HUMAN ANATOMY AND PHYSIOLOGY

# BONE DISORDERS, SCREENING AND TREATMENT

# HUMAN ANATOMY AND PHYSIOLOGY

HUMAN ANATOMY AND PHYSIOLOGY

# BONE DISORDERS, SCREENING AND TREATMENT

AUBREY M. STONE
EDITOR

*New York*

## NOTICE TO THE READER



Additional color graphics may be available in the e-book version of this book.

**Library of Congress Cataloging-in-Publication Data**

ISBN: 978-1-63482-155-1
Library of Congress Control Number: 2015931766

*Published by Nova Science Publishers, Inc. † New York*

# Contents

# Preface

Bone mineral density (BMD) is a determinant of bone health. Phenotype, age, race, gender, activity level and overall health status all affect BMD. Recent research has shown that early pregnancy loss could be associated with bone mineral density. Reduced bone mass, bone density and consequently the pathological conditions, osteopenia and osteoporosis, represent significant health problems and contribute to disability, mortality, and reduced health related quality of life among older women and men. This book examines disorders that affect bone density, such as rickets and osteomalacia, and discusses screening and treatment options available for these and other bone disorders.

Chapter 1 - Bone mineral density (BMD) is one determinant of bone health. Phenotype, age, race, gender, activity level and overall health status all affect BMD. When age and activity level are controlled for, there is a hierarchy of BMD, for Black, Caucasian, and Asian women, respectively. Asians have been shown to have lower areal BMD compared with Caucasians. Paradoxically, the incidence of hip and wrist fractures is lower among Asians. Several authors reported that a significant proportion of young females spend a significant number of their waking hours in sedentary activity. However, the current, collective evidence regarding the historical significance of inactivity on BMD and, by extension, bone health is unknown. Females accrue bone density at a rapid rate during the pubescent year. It follows that inactivity during the pubescent period will have a negative impact on overall bone health, including BMD. Hip fractures are common among the elderly, especially among Caucasians, but these fractures were observed more frequently among females who had not reached the peri and postmenopausal stages of life. According to recent research, the number of hip fractures has declined over the past decade in the United States, however the number of hip and knee arthroplasties is predicted to escalate rapidly over the next 25 years due to osteoarthritis and other joint diseases. If BMD is used as a surrogate for bone health, having healthy bone stock is advantageous to positive patient outcomes following bone surgery. Therefore, the objective of our literature review and systematic review chapter for Bone Mineral Density (BMD):New Research, is to summarize and write a cogent chapter of recent research related to the influence of race on BMD in pre-peri- and post-menopausal females. By extension, the recent literature related to BMD health and the outcomes related to intended and unintended bone insult will be considered. A short list of sub-topics will include: influence of low-grade inflammation on BMD, activity level differences and racial differences among women across three primary time periods, premenopausal, perimenopausal and postmenopausal periods of life.

Chapter 2 - Recent research has shown that pregnancy could be associated be bone mineral density (BMD) loss. The patterns of BMD changes in pregnancy have been evaluated in many recent studies. This BMD loss during the course of pregnancy is largely transient, and should recover within a relatively short period of time in the postpartum period. However, this pregnancy related BMD loss can also become chronic if postpartum recovery fail to occur or was not complete, giving rise to increased risks of osteoporosis in later pre- and post-menopausal life. While radiological methods have been used in the past for monitoring such BMD changes, recent research have shown that the use of quantitative ultrasound for the monitoring of BMD changes in pregnancy is feasible, and is particularly advantageous as it is free from radiation side effects as compared to other standard radiological techniques for BMD measurements, such as dual energy X-ray absorptiometry or quantitative tomography. The use of quantitative USG measurements on different bony sites, including the os calcis or phalanges during pregnancy has been reported and compared. The use of serial quantitative USG has allowed more detailed research into such pregnancy related BMD changes, and significant factors that will influence this change, such as body weight, body fat composition, parity or other antenatal obstetric conditions have been evaluated. Pregnancy symptoms such as low back pain have been associated with BMD changes during pregnancy, while active exercises on the physiological BMD changes during pregnancy have shown that the BMD loss was apparently less compared to those that were not regularly exercising.

Epidemiological data have shown that parity and lactation do not have significant detrimental effects on bone health in later life. This is consistent with the observation that BMD loss during pregnancy and lactation usually recovers within a few years. Overall, pregnancy appears to be a protective or neutral factor against menopausal fractures. The key findings of the current studies would be summarized in this chapter.

Chapter 3 - Obesity and its related comorbidities have long been shown to have detrimental effects on health. Since dietary and lifestyle interventions are often ineffective in producing sustained weight loss, bariatric surgery has become a major therapeutic option for individuals with medically-complicated obesity. Micronutrient disorders including vitamin D deficiency are commonly found in individuals before bariatric surgery, perhaps due to inadequate oral intake of vitamin D or due to vitamin D malabsorption. Vitamin D deficiency has been shown to persist after bariatric surgery. Vitamin D deficiency is a major clinical concern since bariatric patients remain at risk for bone diseases, including osteoporosis and osteomalacia.

Increased pre-operative body mass index has been shown in studies to be a risk factor for vitamin D deficiency. Data regarding different bariatric surgical procedures as risk factors for vitamin D deficiency have been conflicting. It has been suggested that patients who have undergone vertical sleeve gastrectomy or adjustable gastric banding have significantly higher vitamin D levels and improvement in vitamin D deficiency when compared to individuals who have undergone Roux-en-Y gastric bypass. Available results suggest that bariatric procedures which emphasize restrictive strategies may initially improve vitamin D deficiency compared to bariatric procedures which utilize restriction and malabsorption. It has been suggested that the bypass of upper small intestine may promote vitamin D malabsorption. Our studies have however expanded upon prior reports of increased serum levels of folate in individuals with small intestinal bacterial overgrowth. Our results suggest that small intestinal bacterial overgrowth is a potential mechanism to explain post-operative vitamin D deficiency.

Improved understanding of the mechanisms involved in pre-operative vitamin D deficiency and the disorders that inhibit correction of vitamin D deficiency after bariatric surgery should improve the treatment of vitamin D deficiency in individuals who undergo bariatric surgery. Further studies should demonstrate a reduction in the risks of developing osteoporosis and osteomalacia in those individuals who have improved repletion of this important micronutrient.

Chapter 4 - Reduced bone mass, bone density and consequently the pathological conditions osteopenia and osteoporosis represent significant health problems and contribute to disability, mortality, and reduced health related quality of life among older women and men. Consequently the decline of bone mineral content (BMC) and bone mineral density (BMD) are mainly seen as aspects of ageing. Bone loss however may also occur among young people. An important risk factor is low weight status. Especially extreme slenderness in combination with malnutrition such among people suffering from eating disorders may accelerate bone turnover and may result in osteopenia and osteoporosis. The present study examines the impact of weight status – classified by body mass index (BMI) categories defined by the WHO, but also of soft tissue body composition parameters such as body fat and muscle mass on bone mineral content and bone density among 864 Austrian women ageing between 20 and 88 years. Body composition as well as bone density is determined by dual energy x-ray absorptiometry (DXA). A marked impact of weight status and soft tissue body composition on bone density and bone mineral content could be observed for all age groups. This association of low weight status and low bone mass could be proved especially for young women suffering from eating disorders.

Chapter 5 - Regular alcohol consumption is now widespread with public health concerns regarding the effect of excessive intake on all groups. This review considers the relationship between different levels of alcohol intake and bone health among adolescent, pre and post-menopausal women and men, and will discuss the possible mechanisms of alcohol's influence on bone health. In general, regular low levels of alcohol consumption are associated with above average bone mineral density (BMD), while excessive alcohol consumption is associated with reduced BMD possibly through a direct toxic effect on bone turnover but also through associated lifestyle factors.

Chapter 6 - The annual incidence of rickets in the United States is low, at approximately 0.5 per 100,000. This has been achieved largely through vitamin fortification of foodstuffs, primarily dairy products. However, in 2007 one academic primary care clinic located in the eastern portion of the state of South Dakota, whose patient population includes a high proportion of immigrants, experienced an incidence that was 200 times that level. Starting from a discussion of these cases, this chapter reviews the literature regarding rickets and hypovitaminosis D in the upper Midwest region. It discusses specific risks in this population, including environmental factors present in northern climates, physiological factors inherent in subsets of the population, and specific cultural factors, all of which exert significant influences on vitamin D levels and risk of rickets. Prevention, diagnosis, and treatment strategies are presented from the perspectives of primary care of the individual, population health, and public policy.

Chapter 7 - While the bone deformities classically associated with rickets have been recognised for many years, the fact that fractures also occur has been less well appreciated. In fact an association with fractures has been reported since the nineteenth century. This chapter summarises the published reports of fractures in rickets due to vitamin D deficiency. It is clear that fractures often occur spontaneously, may be asymptomatic and may be multiple. While the reported cases were identified because of the finding of radiological evidence of rickets it is important to recognise that rickets may occur without radiological abnormality. Fractures due to rickets are likely to be more frequent than the modest number of cases would suggest. The chapter reviews published reports on fracture risk associated with vitamin D deficiency. It also reviews fractures in forms of rickets not due to vitamin D deficiency and emphasises the differential diagnosis of fractures in young children.

Chapter 8 - Many adults with osteomalacia due to vitamin D deficiency have symptoms for which the underlying cause may not be recognised for months or years. This chapter illustrates the clinical presentations including bone pain, muscle weakness and fractures. It summarises the investigative strategies that are appropriate. It covers the place of clinical examination, of biochemistry, of radiology, of densitometry and of bone biopsy. It also considers the rarer causes of osteomalacia including heritable forms of hypophosphataemia and tumour-induced osteomalacia (oncogenic osteomalacia).

Chapter 9 - Osteomalacia is the equivalent of rickets in the adult and is due to severe, prolonged vitamin D depletion. The diagnosis is challenging and underestimated, but should be considered in patients suffering from proximal muscle weakness, bone pain and a gait disorder that leads to repeated falls. In the following chapter we present the clinical features of osteomalacic myopathy, we discuss current hypothesis about pathogenesis and we show muscle biopsy pictures and EMG recordings of a case recently diagnosed in our Department. Our goal is to make physicians aware of this treatable condition to avoid misdiagnosis.

In: Bone Disorders, Screening and Treatment
Editor: Aubrey M. Stone

ISBN: 978-1-63482-155-1


*Chapter 1*

# Race Influences Bone Mineral Density in Pre-, Peri- and Postmenopausal Females

***William R. Barfield, PhD[1,2], Michael G. Flynn[1], PhD, McKinsey Pratt[1], BS, Meredith Gray[1], BS and Wesley Dudgeon[1], PhD***

[1]Department of Health and Human Performance-College of Charleston-Charleston, SC
[2]Department of Orthopaedics-Medical University of South Carolina-Charleston, SC

## Abstract

Bone mineral density (BMD) is one determinant of bone health. Phenotype, age, race, gender, activity level and overall health status all affect BMD. When age and activity level are controlled for, there is a hierarchy of BMD, for Black, Caucasian, and Asian women, respectively. Asians have been shown to have lower areal BMD compared with Caucasians. Paradoxically, the incidence of hip and wrist fractures is lower among Asians. Several authors reported that a significant proportion of young females spend a significant number of their waking hours in sedentary activity. However, the current, collective evidence regarding the historical significance of inactivity on BMD and, by extension, bone health is unknown. Females accrue bone density at a rapid rate during the pubescent year. It follows that inactivity during the pubescent period will have a negative impact on overall bone health, including BMD. Hip fractures are common among the elderly, especially among Caucasians, but these fractures were observed more frequently among females who had not reached the peri and postmenopausal stages of life. According to recent research, the number of hip fractures has declined over the past decade in the United States, however the number of hip and knee arthroplasties is predicted to escalate rapidly over the next 25 years due to osteoarthritis and other joint diseases. If BMD is used as a surrogate for bone health, having healthy bone stock is advantageous to positive patient outcomes following bone surgery. Therefore, the objective of our literature review and systematic review chapter for Bone Mineral Density (BMD): New Research, is to summarize and write a cogent chapter of recent research related to the influence of race on BMD in pre-peri- and post-menopausal females. By extension, the recent literature related to BMD health and the outcomes related to intended and unintended bone insult will be considered. A short list of sub-topics will include: influence of low-grade inflammation on BMD, activity level differences and racial differences among women across three primary time periods, premenopausal, perimenopausal and postmenopausal periods of life.

# Introduction

Bone mineral density (BMD), as measured with dual-energy X-ray absorptiometry (DXA), is one determinant of bone health. BMD has been used as an independent predictor of fracture risk, especially among peri- and post-menopausal women [6, 7]. Other factors that affect bone health include race, gender, ethnicity, nutritional status, inflammation, activity level and overall health status [8, 26]. Research is published in support of the hierarchy of areal BMD (aBMD) for African American (AA), Caucasian, and Asian women, respectively [9]. However, as will be shown in this literature review, Asians, paradoxically, have a lower incidence of hip and wrist fractures compared with Caucasians [12]. To complicate the issue of aBMD and fracture risk from a predictive perspective, mixed race ethnicity creates additional challenges since aBMD standards for mixed race individuals, used to predict level of bone density/osteoporocity, are not available [44, 70].

The historical significance of inactivity on BMD and, by extension, bone health is not known, but there is strong evidence that a significant proportion of young females spend too many waking hours engaged in sedentary activity. It is well documented that females accrue bone density at a rapid rate during the pubescent years, therefore inactivity, particularly during the pre-teen and early teen years, has a negative impact on overall bone health, including BMD. [5, 126, 139]. At the opposite end of the age spectrum from accruing bone mass in young females, is the risk for hip fractures associated with bone fragility, which is common among the elderly, especially in Caucasian females [8]. Bone insufficiency fractures have also been found among females who have not reached the peri- and post-menopausal stages of life [9]. According to recent research, the number of hip fractures has declined over the past decade in the United States; however, the number of hip and knee arthroplasties (joint replacement) is predicted to escalate rapidly over the next 25 years due to osteoarthritis and other joint diseases [61, 104, 109]. Because BMD is used as a surrogate for bone health, having healthy bone stock is advantageous to positive patient outcomes following bone surgery. Therefore, the objective of our literature review chapter for Bone Mineral Density (BMD): New Research, is to write a cogent chapter summarizing recent research related to the influence of race on BMD in pre-, peri- and post-menopausal females. Recent literature related to BMD health and the outcomes related to intended and unintended bone insult will be considered. We will also address the impact of nutrition, physical activity and low-grade inflammation on BMD in women across three primary time periods; pre-menopausal, peri-menposusal and post-menopausal periods of life.

# BMD Historical Perspective

Historically, aBMD testing was estimated through the use of radiographs. Subsequent findings revealed that x-rays were not sufficiently sensitive and density loss was not apparent until approximately 40% of bone loss had occurred. Over the years, a number of imaging techniques have been used to assess aBMD. Single photon and dual photon absorptiometry (DPA) were used in the 1960's and 1970's; however, the precision was poor and soft tissue distorted the image. Modern aBMD instrumentation allows the quantification of bone mineral content at three locations: distal radius, proximal femur and lumbar spine. These bony locations have a predominance of trabecular bone. Painless, noninvasive, easily performed DXA technology was introduced in the 1980s. DXA uses an x-ray source rather than a radioactive isotope, eliminating the source decay that was a problem with single energy x-ray and DPA. The x-ray source is focused on a single bony/soft tissue area. The proportion of light that passes through, compared with the light that is blocked by minerals, is divided by the surface area of the bone to estimate the aBMD. DXA scan times are short compared with DPA; the radiation dose is very low, in the range of 3 mrem (~10% of the radiation from a normal chest x-ray), and the precision is high (~1-2%) when compared to DPA. A fan-beam scanner, which provides a higher resolution image than a pencil beam scanner, is now employed in most instruments. BMD testing can be used to diagnose bone loss, determine the potential risk of osteopenia and osteoporosis, and predict fracture risk; however, race, sex, menopausal stage all affect the results of a DXA scan [11,103].

> Test results are commonly reported as T-scores and Z-scores. The T-score, the gold standard, is the number of standard deviations above or below the mean for a healthy young woman. Generally, for every standard deviation below normal, the fracture risk doubles. Therefore, if the T-score is two standard deviations below the mean the fracture risk quadruples. The Z score compares an individual's BMD with people of the same gender, age and race. A Z score lower than -1.5 suggests secondary osteoporosis, which means the bone loss is due to something other than age-related osteoporosis [11, 103].

# BMD and Osteoporosis

Osteoporosis (OP) is one of the leading public health issues in the United States, contributing to 1.5 million fractures annually. It has been estimated that 40% of post-menopausal women will have a fracture due to compromised or weakened bone [122].

OP is a debilitating, systemic disease of the skeletal system that decreases a bone's resistance to loads and increases fracture risk due to a reduction in aBMD. OP is a common, worldwide health problem; especially prevalent in developed countries where an estimated 40% of women over the age of 50 [77, 163] are diagnosed with OP.

OP affects more than 75 million women in Europe, Japan and the US. More than a decade ago, OP was believed to contribute to an estimated 2.3 million fractures in Europe and the US [160].

Over a lifetime, women lose about 50% of their trabecular bone and 30% of their cortical bone, with approximately half of the loss occurring during the first 10 years following menopause. Variation in rates of bone loss in the transition to menopause is substantial [37].

A multicenter study examined the aBMD characteristics among 1902 AA, Caucasian, Chinese and Japanese women with a mean age of 46, and an average follow-up of 4 years. Findings showed that aBMD changes little during the pre- and early peri-menopausal period, but declines rapidly late in the peri-menopausal period [16, 17].

Despite these findings, aBMD testing of peri-menopausal women is increasing; but Cauley et al. [23] reported that this may be unnecessary since fracture risk is low in this demographic subgroup. BMD and fracture incidence varies widely across racial and ethnic groups. AA women typically have higher aBMD in axial and appendicular skeletal areas than Caucasians, thereby lowering the incidence of osteoporotic fractures [86, 98, 158]. Asian women have a lower aBMD than Caucasian women, but have a lower rate of fracture, which is a poorly understood phenomenon; although, it appears to be closely tied to anthropometric and mechanical variables (femoral neck width and width) in combination with aBMD [124, 125].

A 2002 study of 2200 women revealed significant differences in aBMD at the lumbar spine and the femoral neck among late pre-menopausal and early peri-menopausal AA, Caucasian, Chinese and Japanese women. The highest BMD was seen in AA women, followed by Caucasian, Chinese and Japanese [44].

Bone deterioration accelerates after menopause due to lower estrogen levels. In a systematic review of 13 studies in which post-menopausal women were subjects, the following factors, previously believed to negatively affect BMD, were inconclusive in predicting low BMD: calcium intake, current and past physical activity, smoking, moderate alcohol consumption (<12 drinks/week), caffeine intake, age of menarche, parity or lactation, history of amenorrhea, family history of OP, race (although only one study in the systematic review studied more than a single race), and age less than 60.

In this review, the factors found to be important in predicting low BMD were: older age (>60), low body weight, and years since menopause [154]. These findings provide evidence of an endocrine effect in older women that is not evident in younger women.

## BMD and Body Mass

Low body weight and ethnicity are believed to be important modifiers of aBMD loss. Therefore, higher body weight is associated with higher aBMD and reduced fracture risk [106,107]. Statistically, body weight accounts for approximately 30% of the variance in aBMD, thereby making body weight one of the strongest predictors of aBMD [56]. One of the unresolved questions in the literature relates to the influence of fat mass and lean mass and their combined and stratified effects on BMD. Some studies suggest that fat mass has the greatest influence [118, 119]. Others suggest that lean mass provides a greater contribution to BMD [60, 63, 152]. In a subsequent section of the chapter, we acknowledge that obesity, especially morbid obesity, and the associated hyper-inflammatory state, may negate some of the body mass effect, due to the potential for the immune system to influence bone.

In 2010, BMD was measured at the femoral neck and lumbar spine in 210 post-menopausal Vietnamese women (mean age 48 years). A statistically significant (p=0.02), but weak correlation (r=0.15) was found between age and percent body fat. Univariate analysis showed lean mass and fat mass both were associated with increased aBMD. Simulated multiple linear regression was used to predict aBMD from a series of independent (predictor) variables and lean body mass was found to be the strongest predictor of aBMD. Lean mass explained 13% of the variance in femoral neck aBMD, whereas fat mass explained 4% of femoral neck aBMD. The lean mass finding suggests that increased physical activity, which is believed to increase lean mass and decrease fat mass, reduces the risk of osteoporosis [60]. The connection between fat and bone is complex because visceral fat, subcutaneous fat, and bone marrow fat all express tissue specific characteristics, and thereby different metabolic properties [80].

In investigations where body weight has been stratified, peri-menopausal and post-menopausal bone loss was significantly slower among AA and Caucasian females compared with Chinese and Japanese women who weighed less [16]. BMD among pre-menopausal and post-menopausal Chinese-American women was influenced by a number of factors including lifestyle. Body weight was a strong predictor of bone density in pre-menopausal and postmenopausal Chinese-American women, accounting for more than 75% of the variance in lumbar spine and proximal femur BMD [148]. The relationship between higher body weight and slower rates of BMD loss is unclear. Osteocytes are known to be sensitive to mechanical loading of bone and may mitigate/minimize the effects of osteoclasts on bone resorption, thereby reducing bone loss [16].

The DXA scanners used to assess BMD may have limited accuracy, which influences the perceived rates of BMD loss. BMD magnitude appears to decrease more slowly in patients with greater subcutaneous fat and higher rates of bone loss are shown with less subcutaneous fat [17]. Rates of spinal aBMD bone loss among AA were slower than that seen among Asians. These differences disappeared when body weight was controlled, indicating that ethnicity was not an independent predictor of bone loss.

## Bone Mineral Density and Fracture Risk

BMD is a reliable predictor of long bone strength and fracture risk [105]. From a quantitative perspective each standard deviation decrease in BMD corresponds to a doubling of overall fracture risk [72]. Patients with low body weight and amenorrhea for more than 3 months should seek appropriate clinical advice to lessen the effect of bone loss [43] due the fact that bone loss is accelerated in the late peri-menopausal period. Vertebral fractures are the most common fracture among older women, estimated at 700,000 annually in the US [25]. Vertebral fractures contribute to the risk of subsequent non-spine fractures and decreased survival [72, 99]. AA women have been found to have approximately half the lifetime fracture risk of Caucasian women; however, these findings are based primarily on non-vertebral fractures [8, 38].

Fragility fracture is defined as a fracture that results from low-impact loading or falling from a standing height, and this fracture is more commonly observed in Caucasian women [21]. A study of fragility fracture risks among four groups of post-menopausal Caucasian,

Asian, AA and Hispanic women, showed that aBMD did not differ between fracture and non-fracture patients [114]. Fractures that resulted from poor bone quality, including fragility fractures, resulted in significant increases in health care dollars spent on treatment [28]. In China and India, the most heavily populated Asian countries, the number of osteopenic and osteoporotic patients is predicted to exceed 300 million by 2020 [4]. In 2012, three post-menopausal ethnic cohorts (South Asian, Chinese and Caucasians) were assessed for aBMD and non-vertebral osteoporotic fractures. Proportional multivariate analyses examined independent predictors for non-vertebral fractures. Prior fracture, lower aBMD, older age, and Caucasian or South Asian race were associated with higher rates of non-vertebral fractures [84].

The prevalence of vertebral fracture has, even in AA women at a younger age has been shown to be 45-50% lower when compared with Caucasian women over the age of 70. Cauley et al., in 2008, showed that volumetric BMD was more strongly associated with vertebral fractures than aBMD at the proximal femur. Based on these findings it appears that bone trabecular number, cortical thickness, and bone remodeling contribute to reduced risk of vertebral and proximal femur fracture in AA women [25].

BMD and proximal femoral measurements were made on 538 Chinese and 788 Caucasian women between the ages of 18-93, living in Australia. Young Chinese women had a shorter femoral neck length, narrower femoral neck width and a thinner femoral neck cortex compared with young Caucasian women. Older Chinese women had a smaller femoral neck periosteal diameter and the neck modulus was lower than among older Caucasian women [151]. Therefore, based on the results of the two previous studies, the value of aBMD measurements of long bone and vertebral fracture risk may present with a different profiles due to bone geometry differences.

Low aBMD, especially at the femoral neck, compared with the lumbar spine and radius, was reported to be an important predictor of fracture risk in women over the age of 65. In this investigation, each age-adjusted standard deviation reduction in femoral neck BMD increased hip fracture risk by 2.6 fold [33]. In 2005, Cauley et al. [23] studied 636 AA and 7334 Caucasian post-menopausal subjects over age 70 for aBMD and fracture risk. AA women were older, weighed more, and had a higher BMI compared with Caucasian women. The incidence of fracture was 30-40% lower among AA women compared to Caucasian women at each site whether BMD was measured areally or by volume [23].

Fracture risk has been shown to be approximately 50% lower among AA women compared with Caucasian women [8,9], the reasons for which are unclear. Higher aBMD among AA women accounts for less than 50% of the variation in fracture risk [44,105], clearly leaving open the possibility that other factors are important. A study of 100 AA and 173 Caucasian women between the ages of 56-66 (93% post-menopausal) showed AA women had greater aBMD (assessed via DXA) at the lumbar spine and proximal femur and higher trabecular volumetric BMD (assessed via HR-pQCT) at the radius and greater cortical tibia thickness. These ethnic differences existed despite lower physical activity levels, higher tobacco use, higher rates of diabetes and hyperthyroidism in the AA women. Thus, it appears that AA women have structural advantages in density and bone microstructure, which likely accounts for lower fracture risk among AA women. [117].

Lower BMD and fracture risk increases with age, although there is significant variation across race/ethnicity [69]. As little as ten years ago, BMD was considered a reliable predictor of hip fracture risk [74]. However, low BMD does not account for racial/ethnic variations in hip fracture risks. For example, Japanese women have lower aBMD than Caucasian women, but have a lower risk of hip fracture [123]. Individual differences within a given racial/ethnic group, such as bone size, genetics, family history and lifestyle make using BMD problematic in estimating fracture risk among some samples and populations [151]. Additionally, there is an incomplete aBMD reference database from which to compare a patient's T and Z scores. Ishii et al., [69] measured BMD on 2,413 women (42-53 years of age) with an intact reproductive system and not using hormone replacement from five ethnic groups (Caucasian, AA, Hispanic, Chinese and Japanese). Three femoral neck bone indices were also used to assess bone strength. Femoral neck aBMD was greatest among AA women, compared to Caucasian, Chinese and Japanese women, respectively. Composite bone strength indices were not significantly correlated with femoral neck aBMD without ethnic stratification. AA, Chinese and Japanese women had higher values on all three strength indices compared with Caucasian women, despite lower aBMD in Japanese and Chinese women. Therefore, composite strength indices that include BMD, femoral neck length, femoral neck width, body weight and height are more useful for accurately predicting racial/ethnic femoral neck bone strength differences among women [69].

Fracture risk has been quantified by clinicians with DXA scans, which provide an areal assessment of bone quality and fracture risk. There are limitations to the predictive accuracy of the DXA scan since BMD does not account for racial and ethnic differences, and therefore does not completely assess fracture risk. Risk assessment is predicated on correct identification of individuals based on race and ethnicity, which is problematic among those of mixed heritage. To this end Ishii et al., in 2012 studied 3302 women between the ages of 42-53 years of age, with at least one ovary, having had at least one menstrual cycle in the last 3 months, and self-identified as Caucasian, AA, Hispanic, Chinese or Japanese. Their aBMD was measured with a DXA scan to determine aBMD at the femoral neck. Three indices were formulated for compression, bending, and impact strength based on the length and width of the femoral neck in combination with weight and height. Femoral aBMD and the three indices for bone strength were inversely associated with fracture risk over 9 years. Race/ethnicity was not predictive of fracture risk independent of the strength indices; however, race/ethnicity improved discrimination in the aBMD based model. Bone strength is a complex combination of race/ethnicity, age, gender, bone geometry, body weight and estimated bone indices. Based on the findings from this study of middle aged women from 5 self-reported races, inclusion of bone indices may be beneficial in predicting fracture risk in women of unknown/mixed and/or un- and under-represented races [70].

The evidence clearly shows that BMD is influenced by bone mass, body composition (as expressed in terms of percentage of lean and fat mass) and race. However, nutritional status has the potential to positively or negatively affect bone mass, body composition and by extension, BMD.

## Bone Mineral Density and Nutrition

It is well established that diet/nutrition can affect several aspects of health status. Nutrition obviously plays a significant role in body composition (muscle mass and fat mass), has the potential to improve mental performance (caffeine), and influence the etiology of chronic diseases such as cancer and cardiovascular disease. Simply put, what we put into our bodies greatly influences how we feel and how we function.

In terms of bone health, the role of diet extends beyond vitamins and minerals, as research has shed light on the negative impacts of other consumables such as smoking, excessive alcohol consumption and low intake of fruits and vegetables. Much of the focus had been on the role of calcium and Vitamin D in bone health, but vitamins A and C and sodium intake have an impact on bone health. In this section of the chapter we will focus on the most studied, and arguably, the most significant nutritional factors related to bone health.

## Calcium

As with the other vitamins and minerals that will be discussed in this section, calcium is essential for many bodily functions, ranging from hormone secretion to skeletal muscle contraction. There is strong evidence showing that adequate consumption of calcium over the lifespan leads to better bone health [108], making calcium the important contributing nutrient for determining bone health [19, 20]. Indeed, adequate calcium intake is required for optimal bone growth and development [68] and impacts the rate of bone loss that occurs with aging. When calcium is under consumed (along with Vitamin D), aberrant hormonal responses result in reduced calcium absorption and increased circulating calcium. The resulting milieu subsequently stimulates parathyroid hormone (PTH) secretion, which leads to increased bone remodeling, and a subsequent loss of bone mass.

Approximately 99% of the body's calcium stores are found in bone and teeth, and bone serves as the primary source of calcium for other needs. The interplay between resorption and deposition of calcium in bones illustrates this point. During times of organismal growth, there is a shift in the favor of bone formation, while later in life, especially in postmenopausal women, there is a decrease in bone deposition and an increase in resorption. Thus, it is important for females to consume recommended doses of calcium (1,000 mg for females over 18 and 1,200 mg for females over 51) [47] early in life to maximize bone mineralization.

Calcium needs extend into the elderly years, as a strong association exists between calcium intake and bone mass in post-menopausal women [58]. Calcium supplementation (500 mg/day) can slow the overall loss of bone by ~1% each year [113], with improvements in hip, [79] spine [155] and forearm bone mass [155].

Evidence exists, even in randomized controlled trials, that calcium supplementation consistently improves bone mass across the lifespan [27, 138, 156]. During pregnancy, the demand for calcium increases due to the increased needs of the fetus. When maternal calcium intake is insufficient calcium is obtained from maternal bone. Only ~20% of women of childbearing age get adequate calcium [144]. During lactation, the infant consumes a significant amount of calcium via the mother's milk, but calcium needs beyond feeding are taken from maternal bone [90].

## Vitamin D

Vitamin D can most accurately be measured in the blood by testing serum 25-hydroxyvitamin [25(OH)D] levels (the result of liver conversion). 25(OH)D has a relatively long half-life, and represents both endogenous vitamin D production and ingestion. Vitamin D performs many vital roles in the body, but germane to bone health is its necessity for calcium absorption. Vitamin D also influences normal osteoclast and osteoblast activity. When dietary calcium is adequate, intestinal absorption is mainly a passive process; however, when calcium levels are low (as is common in most American females) a vitamin D-dependent transport mechanism occurs [19], such that intestinal calcium absorption is increased. In spite of the important relationship between calcium absorption and vitamin D, no definitive guidelines for 25(OH)D levels have been established. The strongest recommendations come from the Institute of Medicine which advocated for a serum level of 50 nmol/L. A level of 50 nmol/L meets the needs (not specific to bone health) of 97.5% of the population. The corresponding Recommended Daily Allowance (RDA) for vitamin D for adult women is 600 IU per day up to age 70, at which time intake should increase to 800 IU [68]. Because of the aforementioned relationship between calcium and Vitamin D, many researchers utilize both substances in their investigations, making it hard to discern the impact of a single nutrient.

Most researchers agree that supplementation with vitamin D alone does not reduce the risk for bone fractures [31]. The verdict is still out, as it was reported that women 69 years or older had a greater risk for frailty when 25(OH)D levels were either low (<50 nmol/L) or high (>75 nmol/L) [25]. There are additional published reports in which a positive relationship was found between serum 25(OH)D levels and bone mineral content [145].

## Sodium

Sodium is an important electrolyte in our diet and is necessary for normal muscle contraction, nerve conduction and the regulation of fluid volume. The recommended intake for sodium is 5,000 mg or less per day. Much of the emphasis on sodium centers on its high consumption in the typical American diet, which, along with other lifestyle choices and susceptibility can increase the risk of, or exacerbate hypertension. This remains a controversial issue, as many of the recommendations for sodium intake are based on research showing that sodium reduction improves blood pressure in those who are already hypertensive; yet, large epidemiological studies in non-hypertensive individuals show no effect of sodium reduction [140].

Adequate sodium intake appears to be important for bone health. The kidneys require that sodium be paired with calcium in order to be excreted in the urine, and studies have shown that high sodium consumption, paired with lower levels of calcium intake, lower bone mass [35], result in elevated PTH levels, and are associated with higher rates of bone resorption in postmenopausal women [57]. Consequently, when sodium intake is reduced, less calcium is excreted and markers of bone turnover reflect improvement [95]. Recently, the key to sodium/calcium relationship has been discovered and we now know that the epithelial sodium/proton (NHE3) exchanger is necessary for the reabsorption of calcium and subsequent excretion of sodium in the intestine and kidneys [113].

## Vitamin C

Collagen is the primary protein found in bone and Vitamin C is necessary for proper collagen synthesis, thus making Vitamin C important for bone health. The National Academy of Sciences recommends adults consume 60-90 mg/day of Vitamin C [47]. There are no clinical control trials assessing the effect of Vitamin C on bone health, but several epidemiological studies suggest a positive relationship between increased Vitamin C consumption and markers of bone health [79, 155].

## Vitamin A

Vitamin A is essential for bone remodeling, mainly by stimulating bone resorption [39]. Vitamin A is consumed in the diet as either retinol (animal sources) or carotenoids (plant sources). The RDA for vitamin A in women is 800 ug/d. An increased risk for impaired bone health may coincide with prolonged intake above 1500 ug/d, as this may interfere with the actions of vitamin D and/or stimulate osteoclast activity. Conversely, elevated carotenoid levels (which also coincide with diets high in fruits and vegetables) have been linked to improved bone health [139]. There have been no clinical controlled trials examining the impact of Vitamin A on bone health, and the observational data is conflicting as some show positive associations [41] and others no relationship between vitamin A and several indices of bone health. [94].

## Smoking

While not a nutritional component, per se, smoking is a lifestyle activity that has long been recognized to impact bone health [34]. Epidemiological work has shown smoking to increase the risk of decreased BMD in young women [13] while post-menopausal women who smoke showed lowered BMD as well [75, 78]. The mechanisms of the impact on bone health are yet to be fully elucidated, but it appears to be a multifactorial etiology with mineral absorption, endocrine function, weight bearing exercise and diet being implicated. Indeed, observational research is consistent in that smoking, regardless of age or other nutritional aspects [78], is deleterious to bone health in a dose-dependent fashion; however, it appears that smoking cessation may partially reverse the damage [162].

## Protein

Approximately half of the mass of the skeletal system is composed of protein, mainly Type I collagen, which cannot be recycled; therefore, new amino acids are constantly needed. Amino acids needed for the synthesis of cellular and extracellular bone proteins [59] stimulate IGF-1, which causes renal production of 25(OH)D and increases tubular inorganic phosphate reabsorption [83]. In stark contrast to reports in the popular media, dietary protein favors calcium absorption and does not result in calcium loss. [29]. Increased protein intake increases urinary calcium, but intestinal calcium absorption also increases [82], resulting in no net loss of calcium. In fact, there is a positive relationship between bone health and protein consumption in pre-menopausal women [32]. Not surprisingly, this relationship extends throughout the life span as a number of studies have shown that higher protein intake is protective against femoral and spinal bone loss [18], and is associated with higher bone density in elderly, hospitalized patients [89]. This evidence has led to the suggestion that protein intake should be increased in the elderly to optimize the environment for bone health [48]. Conversely, some evidence exists to suggest that protein intake below recommendations (0.8 mg/kg/d) can lead to impaired calcium absorption and eventually cause a net loss of calcium from bone [83].

In summary, the research is robust in showing the impact of diet on bone health throughout the lifespan of females of any age and race. From an applied perspective, it appears that women need to maintain an adequate daily intake of protein (0.8 g/kg) while avoiding harmful activities such as smoking. Without a doubt, calcium and vitamin D remain the most important nutritional factors that impact bone health, and because of their interactive nature, it is imperative that both be consumed at adequate levels. Other vitamins (A & C) and minerals (sodium) have a smaller impact on bone health and should be consumed at recommended allowances. Nearly all vitamins and minerals (including those not mentioned in this communication) have the potential to impact bone health. It is therefore critical that females adhere to dietary recommendations during early adulthood to provide the necessary building blocks for bones to grow to full strength, and these healthy habits should remain into later years as proper nutrition can help maintain bone strength.

It is clear that nutritional intake can affect nearly every aspect of human physiology, from endocrine function to bone remodeling, and thus BMD. Yet, there is another lifestyle variable that has the potential to impact most variables that shape BMD; namely physical activity and exercise.

## Exercise and BMD

The positive effects of exercise, both aerobic and anaerobic, on bone health and BMD are generally widely accepted. Current recommendations for improving skeletal health and BMD include all types of training, from aerobic exercises (walking, jogging, and stair climbing) to anaerobic exercises (weight lifting, sprinting, and jumping) to prevent and treat bone loss disorders such as osteopenia and osteoporosis. However, not all exercise modalities are beneficial to bone health, especially when performed in isolation. Furthermore, the efficacy of exercise modalities varies across age groups and is individualized among populations. Therefore, the evidence is inconclusive with regard to the true benefit of all modes of exercise training on bone health throughout the lifespan. Female bone health through pre-, peri- and post-menopausal life phases varies depending on the individual and her stage in life. For instance, rates of bone loss are typically highest in the post-menopausal period, however bone health and rate of loss differs among women based on their lifestyle and overall health. The effect of ethnicity on BMD and bone health is another factor when considering the dose response of physical activity [23].

## Loading Magnitude

The benefits of aerobic exercise in combination with other exercises have been examined in several studies; however, rarely are the benefits of aerobic exercise investigated in isolation. Subsequently, there is little evidence suggesting that aerobic exercise provides a beneficial effect on BMD with the exclusion of all other contributing variables. Most studies showing positive effects of aerobic exercise were observed in specialized populations, in which aerobic exercise should normally elicit favorable BMD changes [50]. These populations include obese pre-/postmenopausal women participating in weight loss programs [62, 120, 121, 133] or osteopenic/osteoporotic females [30, 55, 81, 87]. Thus, when defined to a particular group, aerobic exercise could prove advantageous. In addition, walking is the most common form of aerobic exercise used in testing due to accessibility and low risk. Consequently, the low impact nature of this activity often results in no increase in bone parameters [50]. However, it is important to note that aerobic activity is an effective measure for maintaining or delaying bone loss in postmenopausal older women and may prove more beneficial to bone mass when performed at a higher intensity or when integrated with high impact activities.

The general consensus is that increased bone mass is proportional to the magnitude of the load that is applied through exercise, however there are contrasting positions shown in recent studies. For example, resistance training and high impact activities have produced positive gains in bone mass as a result of the stress applied through mechanical loading. However, studies focused on premenopausal women have found resistance training alone to have no effect on BMD. There are even reports of a negative influence of resistance training when used in combination with aerobic endurance training [3]. Yet, Guadalupe-Grau et al. showed that high intensity aerobic exercises, including jumping and weight training, are essential for improving bone mass in young women [54]. This suggests that combination of both aerobic and anaerobic exercises are necessary to achieve significant benefits. Similarly, Winters-Stone and Snow found that the exercise effects on premenopausal women (aged 33-44) showed increased greater trochanter BMD in response to high impact training, while high impact and resistance training combined increased greater trochanter and lumbar spine BMD [160].

In older postmenopausal women, age appropriate, lower magnitude ground reaction forces (GRF) appear to be important in stimulating the osteogenic response [54]. Kohort et al. studied the effects of GRF (walking, jogging, stair climbing) versus joint reaction forces (JRF) (weight lifting, rowing) on postmenopausal women over a period of 11 months [88]. Both groups experienced BMD increases at the whole body level and femoral neck, however the group that participated in GRF elicited a greater response than the JRF group. Moreover, Chien et al. studied the effect of a 24-week aerobic plus high intensity program on 43 osteopenic postmenopausal women (aged 48-65 years) and found positive BMD improvements at the femoral neck (6.8%) [30]. Exercises included in this study were treadmill walking (aerobic weight bearing exercise) and stepping exercises (high impact exercise) that contributed to strain on the femoral neck, applied 50 minutes, three times per week. These findings suggest that aerobic exercises, in addition to high intensity exercises, may prevent age-related BMD loss. Resistance training can still produce positive effects, but requires higher loading intensities (>70% of 1 RM) with 3-4 sessions per week and 2-3 sets per session [167]. For postmenopausal women, aerobic exercise is probably not sufficient to aid in bone health unless paired with high intensity exercise [54]. In order to preserve BMD in older women and prevent loss of neuromuscular function, high-intensity weight-loading activity should be the primary exercise modality choice.

The best overall exercise prescription to elicit improvements in BMD remains elusive, however, Kemmler et al. found the combination of exercises in a multi-dimensional program to be most effective. An interdisciplinary team including health physicians, sport scientists, and physicians designed an optimal program for preventing bone loss in early postmenopausal women. The study lasted 26 months and involved 137 women (aged 48-60 years). The women were split into an exercise group (n=86) and a control group (n=51). The training program involved a combination of endurance, jumping, strength, and flexibility exercises performed in 4 sessions per week. Results showed that the exercise program was effective for preventing bone loss in the lumbar spine and proximal femur when compared to a significant decrease found in the control group. BMD is impacted through loading magnitude, whereas exercise intensity (strain magnitude) must be greater than minimum strain threshold of bone. This program promoted high-strain rates as well as unusual strain distributions through a wide variety of movements. This finding suggests that prevention of BMD loss is made through key components of each exercise modality rather than one specific type of training [81].

## Resistance Training

Resistance training is often combined with aerobic training when evaluating the effects on BMD and other components of bone health. There are a fairly small number of studies in which resistance training was studied independently. In healthy premenopausal women, it appears resistance training, on its own, does not positively affect BMD, although significant gains in muscle strength have been shown if the stimulus is long enough in duration to illicit positive gains [14, 100]. Mullins and Sinning tested healthy premenopausal women (ages 18-30) taking protein supplements and following the American College of Sports Medicine guidelines for resistance training. Although this study only lasted for 12 weeks, significant increases in muscular strength (25-83% in lower body) were seen; however, there was no increase in BMD [100]. While the reasoning behind why BMD is not improved with resistance training in healthy premenopausal women is unknown, study variables and anatomic locations for BMD change make direct comparisons difficult.

Warren et al. studied a group of overweight, sedentary, premenopausal women (ages 25-44) who were asked to follow the guidelines of the US Department of Health and Human Services for a strength training program for two years. DXA, bone mineral content (BMC) and aBMD were measured at baseline, one year, and two years. BMC was decreased in the femoral neck and no changes were noted in the lumbar spine. Resistance training had no effect on aBMD in either location. The authors concluded that further research is needed on variables that affect BMD which were not captured in this investigation [153]. Laing et al. tested whether upper body exercise affected site-specific increases in BMD among premenopausal women. Following the resistance-training program, there were statistically significant upper body strength gains, but no significant improvement in metabolic markers or BMD of the distal ulna and radius [93].

Peri-menopausal women are the most under researched cohort when assessing the effect of resistance exercise on BMD. The menopausal transition is a time when bone loss is accelerated, yet research on physical activity intervention during this period has not been conducted. Research conducted specifically on women in peri-menopause may shed light on ways to lessen bone loss when transitioning into the postmenopausal stage [135].

The maintenance of BMD in a postmenopausal population is important for reduced fracture risk; therefore, studies with the outcome of preserving BMD should be seen as successful for bone heath in elderly females. Many studies report no change in BMD, however the maintenance of bone health at a time when it is natural to see a reduction should be viewed as a success. In two separate studies, Bocalini et al. [15] and others [50, 54, 55] have studied the effects of moderate intensity (60-70% 1 RM) and high intensity (85% 1 RM) resistance training and found that moderate intensity resistance training resulted in BMD maintenance and high intensity resulted in slight increases of BMD. While the control group had significant reductions in BMD in both the lumbar spine and femoral neck, the training group showed no significant changes in BMD at either the spine or femoral neck [15]. The positive effects of resistance training have been confirmed in similar studies [96, 101, 102, 124].

Strain rate during resistance training has an effect on BMD. Stengal et al. compared strength training (ST) to power training (PT) in osteopenic postmenopausal women. Participants were grouped into ST and PT groups with the difference between the two being the speed of movement. Both groups were involved in supervised resistance training sessions, gymnastic sessions, and at-home training each week. The PT group showed non-significant increases in BMD in both the lumbar spine and the total hip. The ST group demonstrated decreases in BMD in both the lumbar spine and total hip. PT provides higher stresses to the joints leading to the positive effects on BMD. While shown to aid in the maintenance of BMD, higher velocity movement is often avoided in the elderly population due to fears of increased pain. This studied assessed reports of pain and only showed increased reports of neck pain in the PT group. Despite this finding, elderly patients should be monitored during all exercise programs to ensure safety [134].

## Race, Physical Activity, and Bone Mass

Most research examining the effects of exercise on BMD has been conducted on Caucasian populations with limited research on other ethnic populations. Because BMD is positively correlated with higher levels of physical activity (PA), it is of concern that most Americans do not meet the recommended levels of PA. Non-Hispanic black and Hispanic populations, age 60 and older, report lower levels of PA than non-Hispanic Causcasian populations [66].

When studied by Vásquez et al., the trend of all three ethnic/racial groups was correlated with a dose response (higher levels of PA were associated with higher BMD).

However, in the Non-Hispanic AA population, despite the lowest PA levels, there were fewer subjects with osteopenia/osteoporosis. It is speculated that physical activity is not strongly correlated in non-Hispanic AA populations, or that there are factors other than physical activity affecting BMD among this population.

While it is clear that physical activity aids BMD, non-Hispanic AA women have other factors that strongly correlate with their higher levels of BMD [146], including a genetic predisposition to higher levels of BMD compared with other races. Other researchers have confirmed that AA women have lower fracture risk than other ethnicities [23,149]. Despite having the lowest levels of PA, AA postmenopausal women have higher levels of BMD and lower fracture risks [23, 146, 149]. Slower rate of bone loss in AA females may be a contributing factor [24].

## Physical Activity, Body Weight and Fracture Risk

Despite debate on the effect of aerobic exercise on BMD, there is evidence regarding the efficacy of aerobic exercise for lowering fracture risk. Feskanich et al. observed 61,200 postmenopausal women (aged 40-77 years and 98% Caucasian) in 11 US states, beginning in 1986 with a 12 year follow-up [42]. The aim of the study was to examine the effects of walking on hip fracture risk. Fracture risk decreased 6% with each 3-MET- hr/wk of walking. Risk of fracture decreased linearly with exercise intensity increases among women not using hormone replacement. Women who walked at least 4 hrs/week, and were involved in no other forms of exercise, showed a 41% decrease in hip fracture risk.

Moreover, body composition and the effect of exercise plays a significant role in BMD development. Studies of obese post-menopausal women show that BMD tends to decrease with weight loss due to an associated increase in bone resorption [120, 121]. Silverman et al. studied the effects of aerobic exercise combined with a hypo caloric diet on overweight postmenopausal women during a 6-month period. Their exercise/diet protocol resulted in an increase in $VO_{2max}$, increase in femoral neck BMD, and a corresponding decrease in inflammatory markers. Thus, the reduced inflammatory response following weight loss, in addition to improved fitness, could potentially result in increased BMD [131]. Similarly, Hosny et al. [24] studied the impact of aerobic exercises on obese premenopausal women under caloric restriction. Forty women (aged 30-40 years) participated in the study over 3 months. They were separated into 2 groups; one received a restricted caloric diet while the other received restricted caloric diet combined with aerobic exercise. The group that combined a restricted diet and aerobic exercise showed increased BMD of weight bearing bones (L2-L4 and total hip) [62]. There was a significant decrease in BMD of the radius for both groups, which may have been due to lack of upper extremity exercises. Overall, these findings show positive effects of aerobic exercise on BMD, in both pre and postmenopausal women particularly related to overweight/obese individuals undergoing weight loss. Low BMD in premenopausal women is a major determinant for future osteoporotic fractures, and weight bearing activities (walking) are most commonly prescribed for prevention [112].

Swimmers' participation in a reduced gravity activity will obtain less skeletal benefits than those who participate in weight bearing activities that apply mechanical stress to bones [138].

Regardless of comparisons between aerobic activities, research has shown positive impacts of aerobic exercise on BMD, and physically active individuals have higher BMD than those who are sedentary. Andreoli et al. conducted a retrospective study to determine the effects of being involved in sports during youth on BMD, and whether these effects persisted through menopause [3]. A total of 48 Caucasian women (aged 54-73 years) were divided into 3 groups: swimmers (n=12), runners (n=12), and non-athletes (n=24) to serve as the control group. Activity levels over the past 15 years were recorded, as well as activity level at the time of the study. Measurements of BMD, BMC, fat mass and lean mass were recorded using DXA. When athletes were stratified between weight bearing and non-weight bearing sports, runners had significantly higher leg BMD than swimmers. The most significant differences were found when athletes were compared with sedentary controls, which suggests that weight bearing activities, whether weight bearing or buoyancy based, leads to beneficial increases in BMD. Athletes had significantly higher BMD and BMC compared to sedentary controls of similar age and menopausal status. There were not significant differences between swimmers and runners. These findings show that physical activity during youth has beneficial effects on bone mass in later age. In addition, the type of physical activity performed is not specific to weight bearing; that is, both weight bearing and non-weight bearing exercises performed during youth induce positive changes in bone mass that persist through aging [3].

Using a slightly different approach Winters and Snow studied the detraining effects of exercise on premenopausal women. Forty-one women (aged 30-45 years) participated in a 12-month high-impact plus resistance-training program, followed by a subsequent 6-month detraining program. The program consisted of 100 jumps and 100 repetitions of resistance training exercises performed 3 times a week. After the 12-month training program, exercisers had significantly greater BMD values at the greater trochanter, femoral neck, and whole body. In addition, there were improvements in lower extremity strength, power, and body composition. After 6-months of detraining, BMD values, muscle strength, and power all returned to baseline values. These declines indicate reversibility of exercise effects on the musculoskeletal system. Thus, although high-intensity plus resistance- training produces positive effects on BMD, strength, and power in premenopausal women, these effects are reversed with the removal of exercise. This illustrates a positive linear relationship between exercise and musculoskeletal improvements, suggesting that continued training is required to maintain the musculoskeletal benefits achieved through exercise [159, 160].

The robust data linking exercise and BMD suggests this lifestyle choice has a multifactorial impact on bone health. Additionally, the recent literature is ripe with research linking physical activity to systemic inflammation. Thus, we will next examine the relationship between inflammation and bone.

## Bone Mineral Content and Inflammation

Among the many possible factors contributing to a loss of BMD, the role of low-grade systemic inflammation, sometimes called sterile inflammation, in bone loss is relatively new and somewhat controversial. Inflammatory biomarkers were linked to indices of bone-density roughly two decades ago [73, 168], initially with an association between rheumatoid arthritis and other inflammatory diseases and bone losses [147].

More recent research illustrates the importance of the inflammation-inducing toll-like receptor ligation, NFκB activation, and subsequent activation of osteoclasts and promotion of osteoporosis. Specifically, removing a "governor" of the inflammatory signaling pathways resulted in mice developing severe osteoporosis. This bone loss was due to a lack of IRAK-M (IL-1 receptor-associated kinase M), which slows downstream signaling from toll-like receptors and other inflammation inducing ligands [92]. Thus, a strong link between inflammatory processes and bone losses is emerging in the literature.

There are racial differences in inflammatory biomarkers [40] leading to the conclusion that inflammation-linked diseases are higher in AA compared with Caucasians. However, the differences are opposite from what would be expected.

That is, AA appears to have higher levels of inflammatory biomarkers, but also tend to have higher BMD. We will address this apparent contradiction later in this section of the chapter.

Overall, in this section we will discuss the influence of inflammatory cytokines on bone, influence of inflammation and inflammatory signaling on osteogenesis, racial differences in inflammatory markers, the anti-inflammatory effects of exercise, and the obesity paradox.

## Inflammatory Cytokines and Bone

Early research, in which inflammatory biomarkers were linked to bone, was generally observational or correlational. As an example, Cauley et al. [22] reported that several inflammatory biomarkers, such as C-reactive protein (CRP), interleukin-6 (IL-6), and tumor necrosis factor-α (TNF-α) were linked to increased fracture rates in a population of 2985 older Caucasian and AA (42%) men and women (51%). In fact, Cauley et al [22] showed a progressive increase in fracture rate with inflammation, such that those with three or more inflammatory markers in the highest quartile had a relative fracture risk 2.65-fold (CI-1.44-4.89) higher than subjects with zero inflammatory marker levels in the upper quartile. Researchers have also used molecular biology techniques, or examined select aspects of signaling pathways, to illustrate the connection between inflammation-inducing receptors/pathways, osteoclast activation and bone loss [71, 92]. Finally, there is a strong association between bone loss and chronic inflammatory diseases such as rheumatoid arthritis, ankylosing spondylitis, Crohn's disease, and lupus erythematosus. Several of these diseases are treated with anti-inflammatory antibodies, such as anti-TNF-α or anti-IL-6 therapies, which are now used to treat osteoporosis [142].

C-reactive protein is a marker of low-grade systemic inflammation and has been reported to be a strong, independent predictor of fracture risk [127]. Schett et al. followed a cohort of 919 patients from Bruneck, Italy through periodic exams (every five years) to a 20-year follow-up. The subjects were followed for over 3500 person years per tertile. There was a progressively higher non-traumatic fracture incidence in the low (5 fractures), medium (14 fractures), and high (50 fractures) tertiles for CRP [127]. These findings were supported by the work of Cauley et al. [22] and Amadi-Abhari et al. [1], but the latter group reported an unusual, U-shaped relationship between CRP and fracture rate. In their study of 18,586 subjects in the EPIC (European Prospective Investigation into Cancer) Ahmadi-Abhari et al. [1] compared broad age range (40-70) of subjects and had over 260,000 person years of follow up. Total fracture rate was significantly higher in the upper quintiles for CRP, but also in the lowest quintile for CRP. Thus, while fracture rates were linked to high levels of a marker for sterile inflammation, the increased fracture risk in those with the lowest CRP is difficult to explain.

Other researchers who reported a relatively weak relationship between CRP and either bone density or fracture risk offered neutrophil-to-lymphocyte ratio (N:L) as an alternative marker. Yilmaz et al. [166] reported that both N:L and CRP were elevated in a group of osteoporotic women compared to osteopenic women and control group women, but significant correlations were observed only between N:L and lumbar spine BMD. No significant relationships were found between CRP and measures of BMD. Findings of marginal predictive ability of CRP and bone loss were supported by other researchers [110]. Despite some variations in the markers used, and a lack of clearly consistent findings in the literature, it appears that a range of inflammatory biomarkers have been used to predict fracture risk or low BMD. Collectively, there is strong evidence of inflammation and immune cells having deleterious effects on bone, but the strength of relationships between BMD and selected inflammatory biomarkers is inconsistent. As a testament to the fact that there is consistent evidence of a bone-inflammation connection, a new phrase was coined to capture the essence of the relationship between bone, inflammation, and immune function—osteoimmunology [76].

## Influence of Inflammation and Inflammatory Signaling on Osteogenesis

Toll-like receptors are inflammation-inducing receptors, which react to a variety of extracellular pathogens such as the bacterial cell wall-associated lipopolysaccharide (LPS), and viral DNA. LPS elicits a strong external stimulus for bone loss. As mentioned briefly earlier in this section of the chapter, IRAK-M is analogous to a brake or governor for the downstream signaling pathway for the toll-like receptors [92]. TLR signaling activates the downstream pathway, terminating in the activation of the transcription factor NFκB, which up-regulates inflammatory cytokine transcription and activates other aspects of innate immunity. Therefore, IRAK-M tempers TLR signaling and an absence of IRAK-M allows the unrestrained downstream signaling processes, resulting in activation of NFκB and other signaling proteins (p38, JNK, ERK). Therefore, in cells lacking IRAK-M, TLR signaling and NFκB activation would proceed unabated [92]. LPS triggers inflammatory bone loss through TLR4 signaling and TLR4 signaling also promotes osteoclastogenesis [71]. Therefore, the absence of IRAK-M would be predicted to promote osteoclastogenesis and bone loss. Indeed, Li et al. [92] found that IRAK-M knockout mice had rampant osteoporosis, apparently secondary to increased activation and an extended half-life of osteoclasts. These findings help to illustrate the importance of the regulation of inflammatory pathways and the prevention of hyper-inflammatory states caused by morbid obesity, sedentariness, or advanced age.

Activation of selected inflammatory pathways is clearly detrimental to bone. It follows that nutritional or pharmacological strategies designed to suppress inflammation would ameliorate inflammation-associated bone losses. To this end, Huang et al. [64] treated ovariectomized mice with myricitrin, a botanical flavonal glycoside with anti-inflammatory, anti-oxidant and other bio-active properties. Peroxide ($H_2O_2$) treatment of these ovariectomized mice stimulated oxidative injury, increased IL-6 and RANKL (receptor activator of nuclear factor kappa beta, NFκB), and exacerbated trabecular bone loss, all of which were blunted by myricitrin treatment. That is, inhibiting oxidative damage and the resultant inflammatory signaling, spared bone loss in estrogen deficient animals.

As mentioned above, a class of drugs with anti-TNF-α (or anti-IL-6) antibodies is employed in the pharmacological treatment of several chronic diseases. These drugs are used to treat rheumatoid arthritis, ankylosing spondylitis, Crohn's disease and other chronic inflammatory diseases, all of which are also associated with significant bone loss. As an example, anti-TNF-α monoclonal antibodies (e.g., infliximab) are used as one of a class of several drugs in the treatment of rheumatoid arthritis. Since these drugs are effective in the treatment of chronic inflammatory diseases, it follows that osteoporosis may be prevented or reversed by drug treatment.

The use of anti-inflammatory antibodies in the treatment of osteoporosis is relatively new, but evidence exists to support the contention that these drugs are helpful in preserving bone. For example, anti-TNF therapy was reported to increase bone density in patients with spondyloarthritis [36]. Durnez et al. reported an ~12% increase in lumbar spine BMD after a six-year follow-up in a small study group of spondyloarthritis patients (n=59) taking anti-TNF-α drugs, compared to the control group. To the contrary, Timmen et al. [142] found that anti-TNF-α therapy provided some benefit to transgenic mice (hTNFtg) that develop a chronic inflammatory arthritis, but these authors stopped short of concluding that there was am enhanced rate of repair of induced femoral fractures.

Preventing NFκB activation using anti-RANKL antibodies provides another alternative for treating inflammatory diseases and preventing associated bone losses. Anti-RANKL (denosumab) was discovered roughly two decades ago and was approved for use as a treatment for osteoporosis in Europe and the US in 2010 and Japan in 2013 [165]. Use of denosumab and other anti-resorptive agents is gaining traction in the treatment of bone loss and provides an alternative to bisphosphates and other drug therapies. Poole et al. [116] randomized 80 women with osteoporosis into a clinical trial with either twice-yearly denosumab or placebo. The denosumab-treated group had significant increases in femoral cortical mass after only 12 months, ending with a 5.4% increase after three years. Thus, the use of inflammation blocking, anti-resorptive drugs has a promising future in the treatment of both chronic inflammatory diseases and osteoporosis.

## Racial Differences in Inflammatory Biomarkers

As discussed elsewhere in this chapter, AA tend toward higher BMD than Caucasians or Asians. Based on the links between inflammation and bone presented above, a similar hierarchy of race and inflammatory biomarkers would be expected, with AA, Caucasians, and Asians having lowest, moderate, and highest inflammatory biomarkers, respectively. However, the information gleaned from the literature does not provide clear-cut information on racial differences in inflammatory biomarkers and the available evidence runs counter to what would be expected. That is, there is evidence that inflammatory biomarkers are higher in AA [40], but AA often have higher bone density, making it possible that other factors linked to bone accretion supersede the inflammatory mechanisms outlined above.

There is evidence of elevated inflammatory biomarkers in persons of African ancestry compared to those of European ancestry [40, 85, 111], yet the evidence is conflicting. For example, Paalani et al. [111] found that that CRP and IL-6 were significantly higher in African ancestry subjects, but the CRP differences disappeared when socio-economic, dietary and exercise factors were controlled. Engaging in exercise and vegetarian diet were also associated with lower CRP levels. Moreover, there were no baseline differences for TNF-α and IL-10 (anti-inflammatory cytokine) between these racial groups. Several studies can be cited that lend credence to the premise that there may be racial differences in inflammatory biomarkers [2,150]. For example, Anand et al. [2] observed a significantly higher CRP in Asian and Aboriginal subjects, compared to European ancestry subjects when comparing over 1200 subjects from Hamilton, Toronto, and Edmonton, Canada. There is also evidence that differences in inflammatory biomarkers are linked to genetic markers. Thus, they may be linked to different proportion of SNPs (single nucleotide polymorphisms) among races, with the strongest association between SNPs for CRP and CRP plasma concentrations [150].

Chronic hyperglycemia results in elevated blood and tissue concentrations of advanced glycation end products (AGEs). Advanced glycation end products are "senescent macro protein derivatives" which cause damage, oxidant stress, NFκB activation and are linked to several chronic diseases and disease complications [164]. However, high circulating levels of sRAGE (soluble receptor for AGE) are related to reduced disease risk, likely due to sRAGEs ability to adsorb the potentially damaging AGEs. Selvin et al. [129] compared sRAGE levels and disease/mortality risk in over 1200 subjects in the ARIC (atherogenic risks in communities) study. The lowest quartile for sRAGE had the highest number of AA, males, diabetics, hypertensive subjects and the highest CRP levels. Moreover, the low sRAGE quartile had hazard ratios that were significantly higher for all-cause mortality and separate racial analysis showed that AA were three times more likely to have low sRAGE. Other authors reporting racial differences in inflammatory biomarkers had findings conflicting with the premise that inflammation is higher in AA. Whelton et al. [157] compared (n=6735) Caucasian, AA, Chinese, and Hispanic subjects in their MESA study (Multi-Ethnic Study of Atherosclerosis) with the intent of linking resting heart rate to inflammatory biomarkers. Elevated heart rate is linked to adverse cardiac events and these authors linked the known atherogenic and plaque destabilizing risks of inflammation with higher resting heart rate and higher sympathetic outflow. However, there were no differences in response between racial groups in this study.

There is evidence of racial differences in inflammatory biomarkers, but there are some conflicting data. Nevertheless, arriving at a conclusion of elevated inflammation in AA provides a conundrum when making the argument that inflammation is linked to bone loss. There is some evidence of higher inflammatory biomarkers in Asians, which might explain higher incidence of osteoporosis in the Asian population. However, in the same study, persons of Chinese descent had lower CRP than persons of European origin [2]. Bone loss mechanisms appear to be stimulated by inflammation, but inflammatory markers, per se, do not appear to explain racial differences in BMD.

## Anti-Inflammatory Effects of Exercise

Dynamic physical activity generally promotes bone accretion. In addition, exercise training or high levels of physical activity have been clearly shown to elicit anti-inflammatory effects. If bone loss/accretion is indeed linked to inflammatory status, the ability of exercise to positively influence bone could be linked in part, to these anti-inflammatory mechanisms. Exercise has been shown to elicit anti-inflammatory effects in muscle [53,91], adipose tissue [65], LPS-stimulated whole blood cultures [46, 115, 133], and serum [133]. The anti-inflammatory changes do not appear to be exercise mode specific, as we found exercise training exerted anti-inflammatory effects following resistance training [115], combined resistance and aerobic training [143], and in individuals who were simply identified as being highly physically active [97]. There are reports that home-based exercise did not produce measurable anti-inflammatory effects [10]. The lack of effect of home-based programs brings in the possibility that compliance was low and opens the possibility that there is a minimum threshold for exercise training to induce improvements. Nevertheless, the threshold for anti-inflammatory improvements is attainable as a resistance training program of only three days per week (three sets, ten exercises, 80% 1RM) elicited an anti-inflammatory effect [115].

Earlier in this section, toll-like receptor signaling was identified as a potent stimulator of osteoclasts and that accelerated TLR signaling induced osteoporosis [71, 91]. After finding that lipopolysaccharide (LPS)-stimulated inflammatory cytokine production was blunted by 10 weeks of resistance training [115], we sought to determine whether the cell-surface receptor for LPS, toll-like receptor 4 (TLR4), would be influenced by exercise training. We found that TLR4 mRNA was reduced after resistance training in elderly women [46]; that monocyte-surface TLR4 was significantly lower in physically active elderly women compared to age-matched sedentary women [97]; and that 12 weeks of resistance training substantially reduced TLR4 receptor expression on monocytes [133].

Despite the TLR4 suppressing actions of exercise and the known influence of TLR4 signaling on bone, a direct link between exercise training-induced TLR4 reduction and bone accretion has not been elucidated. However, exercise-related mechanisms for bone accretion are typically bone loading and linked to GRFs or muscle forces acting on bone. Exercise-induced suppression of inflammation provides another possible link for the positive influences of exercise on bone.

### The Obesity Paradox—Does Inflammation Play a Role?

Obesity was generally believed to provide an advantage for maintaining bone health [5], in part due to increased mechanical loading. More recently, the generalized hyper-inflammatory state linked to obesity and other metabolic and endocrine factors have been considered, leading to the possibility that an increased fracture risk occurs with increased adiposity [45]. The tipping point between additional fat weight promoting bone health or bone losses may lie in the severity of the obesity and in the visceral fat volume. Greco et al. [52] studied obese women (35.8 kg/m$^2$ BMI) and found a substantial subgroup (37%) that had a lower than expected lumbar BMD. When all subjects (n=398) were sub grouped based on BMI, the overweight subjects (BMI 25-29.9) appeared to be protected from bone loss while the obese group (BMI > 30) had evidence of osteoporosis. Thus, while the historical perspective was that obesity is compatible with bone health, extreme obesity, especially obesity combined with advanced age and estrogen deficiency, could abolish any protective effect associated with higher fat mass [130].

Visceral fat is linked with a high risk of several diseases and is an aggressive producer of inflammatory cytokines. Exercise training selectively targets visceral fat and there are several reports of exercise-training induced reductions in visceral fat, even when the total body fat levels are not significantly affected [49, 67, 132, 141]. Thus, both endurance and resistance exercise provide a means to reduce this potentially harmful adipose depot or reduce the harmful effects by inducing a generalized anti-inflammatory milieu. Obese individuals who undertake a modest program of regular exercise may regain the body mass advantage for bone growth that was previously believed to exist.

## Conclusion

It is clear that maintaining BMD across the lifespan is a significant health issue for women of all ethnicities. The causes for low BMD range from hormonal changes, to dietary factors, to physical activity (and exercise) and even include systemic inflammation. To complicate the picture even further, these variables interact with one another such that physical activity levels can influence inflammation, hormonal changes can in turn influence inflammatory levels and dietary factors can influence all the above. Further, it is apparent that variations in bone health exist among ethnicities, and the response of these groups to changes in the variables that impact BMD may differ. This poses a challenge to researchers and clinicians to better understand the racial differences in relation to BMD in women, especially given that many at risk populations are being underrepresented in existing literature. Finally, it is imperative that women of all ages and ethnicities focus on the entire scope of factors that influence BMD, and not just on modifying one variable in expectation of seeing tangible changes.

## References

[1] Ahmadi-Abhari, S., Luben, R.N., Wareham, N.J., Khaw, K.T. (2013). C-reactive protein and fracture risk: European prospective investigation into cancer norfolk study. *Bone,* 56(1), 67-72.

[2] Anand, S. S., Razak, F., Yi, Q., Davis, B., Jacobs, R., Vuksan,V., Lonn, E., Teo, K., McQueen, M., Yusuf, S. (2004). C-reactive protein as a screening test for cardiovascular risk in a multiethnic population. *Arteriosclerosis Thrombosis and Vascular Biology*, 24(8), 1509-1515.

[3] Andreoli, A., Celi, M., Volpe, S., Sorge, R., Tarantino. U. (2012). Long-term effect of exercise on bone mineral density and body composition in post-menopausal ex-elite athletes: a retrospective study. *European Journal of Clinical Nutrition*, 66(1), 69-74.

[4] Asian Audit (2009). Epidemiology, costs and burden of osteoporosis in Asia 2009. *International Osteoporosis Foundation.*

[5] Baharudin, A., Zainuddin, A.A., Manickam, M.A., Ambak, R., Ahmad, M.H., Naidu, B.M., Cheong, S.M., Ying, C.Y., Saad, H.A., Ahmad, N.A. (2014). Factors associated with physical inactivity among school-going adolescents:data from the Malaysian school-based nutrition survey 2012. *Asian Pacific Journal of Public Health*, 26, 27S-35S.

[6] Barfield, W. R., Calandra, J. J., Hayes, M., Coker, P., Calandra, K. R., Johnson, K. (2014). Comparison of immature porcine and human bone mineral density about the knee:implications for graft pullout studies. *Current Orthopaedic Practice*. 25(2), 147-151.

[7] Barfield, W. R, Otteni, J. F, McBryde, A. M, Carter, J. S, Nietert, P. J. (2005). Longitudinal study of factors affecting stress fracture risk in two distinct college female populations. *Journal of Exercise and Sport Science*, 1(1), 29-41.

[8] Baron, J. A., Barrett, J., Malenka, D., Fisher, E., Kniffin, W., Bubolz, T., Tosteson, T. (1994). Racial differences in fracture risk. *Epidemiology*, 5, 42-47.

[9] Barrett-Connor, E., Siris, E. S., Wehren, L. E., Miller, P. D., Abbott, T. A., Berger, M. L., Santora, A. C., Sherwood, L. M. (2005). Osteoporosis and fracture risk in women of different ethnic groups. *Journal of Bone and Mineral Research*, 20, 185-194.

[10] Beavers, K. M., Brinkley, T.E., B. J. Nicklas, B. J. (2010). Effect of exercise training on chronic inflammation. *Clinica Chimica Acta,* 411(11-12), 785-793.

[11] Berry, S. D., Samelson, E. J., Pencina, M. J., McLean, R. R., Cupples, L.A., Broe, K. E., Kiel, D. P. (2013). Repeat bone mineral density screening and prediction of hip and major osteoporosis fracture. *Journal of the American Medical Association,* 310, 1256-1262.

[12] Bhudhikanok, G. S., Wang, M. C., Eckert, K., Matkin, C., Marcus, R., Bachrach, L.K. (1996). Differences in bone mineral in young Asian and Caucasian American may reflect differences in bone size. *Journal of Bone and Mineral Research*, 11, 1545-1556.

[13] Blair, S. N., Cheng, Y., Holder, J. S. (2001). Is physical activity or physical fitness more important in defining health benefits? *Medicine & Science in Sport and Exercise*, 33 (6 Suppl), S379-399; discussion S419-320.

[14] Blimkie, C. J. R., Rice, S., Webber, C. E., Martin, J., Levy, D., Gordon, C. L. (1996). Effects of resistance training on bone mineral content and density in adolescent females. *Canadian Journal of Physiology and Pharmocology*, 74(9), 1025-1033.

[15] Bocalini, D. S., Serra, A. J., Santos, L. D. (2010). Moderate resistance training maintains bone mineral density and improves functional fitness in postmenopausal women. *Journal of Aging Research*, 2010, 760-818.

[16] Bolotin, H. H. (2001). Inaccuracies inherent in dual x-ray absorptiometry in vivo bone mineral densitometry may flaw osteopenic/osteoporotic interpretations and mislead assessment of antirespoptive therapy effectiveness. *Bone,* 28, 548-555.

[17] Bolotin, H. H., Sievanen, H., Grashuis, J. L. (2003). Patient-specific DXA bone mineral density inaccuracies: quantative effects of nonuniform extraosseous fat distributions. *Journal of Bone and Mineral Research*, 18, 1020-1027.

[18] Broe, K. E., Hannan, M. T., Kiely, D. K., Cali, C. M., Cupples, L.A., Kiel, D.P. (2000). Predicting fractures using bone mineral density: a prospective study of long-term care residents. *Osteoporosis International,* 11 (9), 765-771.

[19] Cashman, K. (2003). Prebiotics and calcium bioavailability. *Current Issues in Intestinal Microbiology*, 4 (1), 21-32.

[20] Cashman, K. D. (2007). *Calcium and vitamin D. Novartis Foundation Symposium,* 282, 123-138, discussion 138-142, 212-128.

[21] Cauley, J. A. (2011). Defining ethnic and racial differences in osteoporosis and fragility fractures. *Clinical Orthopaedics and Related Research,* 469, 1891-1899.

[22] Cauley, J. A., Danielson, M.E., Boudreau, R. M., Forrest, K. Y., Zmuda, J. M., Pahor, M., Tylavsky, F. A., Cummings, S.R., Harris, T. B., Newman, A.B., Health, A., B., C., S. (2007). Inflammatory markers and incident fracture risk in older men and women: the Health Aging and Body Composition Study. *Journal of Bone and Mineral Research.* 22(7), 1088-1095.

[23] Cauley, J. A., Lui, L. Y., Ensrud, K. E., Zmuda, J. M., Stone, K. L., Hochberg, M.C., Cummings, S.R. (2005). Bone mineral density and the risk of incident nonspinal fractures in black and white women. *Journal of the American Medical Association,* 293(17), 2012-2018.

[24] Cauley, J.A., Lui, L.Y., Stone, K.L. Hillier, T.A., Zmuda, J.M., Hochberg, M., Beck, T.J., Ensurd, K.E. (2005). Longitudinal study of changes in hip bone mineral density among Caucasian and African-American Women. *Journal of the American Geriatrics Society*, 53(2), 183-189.

[25] Cauley, J. A., Palermo, L., Vogt, M., Ensrud, K. E., Ewing, S., Hochberg, M., Nevitt, M. C., Black, D.M. (2008). Prevalent vertebral fractures in black women and white women. *Journal of Bone and Mineral Research*, 23, 1458-1467.

[26] Cauley, J. A., Parimi, N., Ensrud, K. E., Bauer, D.C., Cawthon, P.M., Cummings, S. R., Hoffman, A. R., Shikany, J.M., Barrett-Connor, E., Orwoll, G. (2010). Osteoporotic fractures in men's research. serum 25-hydroxyvitamin D and the risk of hip and nonspine fractures in older men. *Journal of Bone Mineral Research*, 25 (3), 545-553.

[27] Chee, W. S., Suriah, A. R., Chan, S. P., Zaitun, Y., Chan, Y. M. (2003). The effect of milk supplementation on bone mineral density in postmenopausal Chinese women in Malaysia. *Osteoporosis International,* 14 (10), 828-834.

[28] Cheng, S. Y., Levy, A. R., Lefaivre K. A., Guy, P., Kuramoto, L., Sobolev, B. (2011). Geographic trends in incidence of hip fractures: a comprehensive literature review. *Osteoporsis International*, 22, 2575-2586.

[29] Chevalley, T., Rizzoli, R., Hans, D., Ferrari, S., Bonjour, J.P. (2005). Interaction between calcium intake and menarcheal age on bone mass gain: an eight-year follow-up study from prepuberty to postmenarche. *Journal of Clinical Endocrinology and Metabolism*, 90 (1), 44-51.

[30] Chien, M. Y., Wu, Y. T., Hsu, A. T, Yang, R.S., Lai, J.S. (2000). Efficacy of a 24-week aerobic exercise program for osteopenic postmenopausal women. *Calcified Tissue International*, 67 (6), 443-448.

[31] Chung, M., Balk, E. M., Brendel, M., Ip, S., Lau, J., Lee, J., Lichtenstein, A., Patel, K., Raman, G., Tatsioni, A., Terasawa, T., Trikalinos, T. A. (2009). Vitamin D and calcium: a systematic review of health outcomes. *Evidence Report/Technology Assessment* (Full Rep)(183), 1-420.

[32] Cooper, C., Atkinson, E. J., Hensrud, D. D., Wahner, H. W., O'Fallon, W. M., Riggs, B.L. Melton, L. J.3rd (1996). Dietary protein intake and bone mass in women. *Calcified Tissue International*, 58 (5), 320-325.

[33] Cummings, S. R., Black, D. M., Nevitt, M. C., Browner, W., Cauley, J., Genant, H. K., Palermo, L., Scott, J., Vogt, T.M. (1993). Bone density at various sites for prediction of hip fractures. The Study of Osteoporotic Fractures Research Group. *Lancet*, 341, 72-75.

[34] Daniell, H. W. (1976). Osteoporosis of the slender smoker. Vertebral compression fractures and loss of metacarpal cortex in relation to postmenopausal cigarette smoking and lack of obesity. *Archives of Internal Medicine*, 136 (3), 298-304.

[35] Devine, A., Criddle, R.A., Dick, I.M., Kerr, D.A., Prince, R.L.(1995). A longitudinal study of the effect of sodium and calcium intakes on regional bone density in postmenopausal women. *American Journal of Clinical Nutrition,* 62 (4), 740-745.

[36] Durnez, A., Paternotte, S., Fechtenbaum, J., Landewe, R. B., Dougados, M., C. Roux, C., Briot, K. (2013). Increase in bone density in patients with spondyloarthritis during anti-tumor necrosis factor therapy: 6-year followup study. *Journal of Rheumatology*. 40(10), 1712-1718.

[37] Falch, J. A., Sandvik, L. (1990). Perimenopausal appendicular bone loss: a 10-year prospective study. Bone, 11, 425-428; Hansen, M.A., Overgaard, K., Riis, B., Christiansen, C. (1991). Role of peak bone mass and bone loss in postmenopausal osteoporosis: 12-year study. *British Medical Journal*, 303, 961-964.

[38] Farmer, M.E., White, L.R., Brody, J. A., Bailey, K.R. (1984). Race and sex differences in hip fracture incidence. *American Journal of Public Health,* 74, 1374-1380.

[39] Fell, H. B., Mellanby, E. (1952). The effect of hypervitaminosis A on embryonic limb bones cultivated *in vitro*. *Journal of Physiology*, 116 (3), 320-349.

[40] Ferguson, J. F., Patel, P.N., Shah, R. Y., Mulvey, C. K., Gadi, R., Nijjar, P.S., Usman, H.M., Mehta, N. H., Shah, R., Master, S.R., Propert, K. J., Reilly, M.P. (2013). Race and gender variation in response to evoked inflammation. *Journal of Translational Medicine*, 11, 63.

[41] Feskanich, D., V. Singh, W. C. Willett and G. A. Colditz (2002). Vitamin A intake and hip fractures among postmenopausal women. *Journal of the American Medical Association*, 287 (1), 47-54.

[42] Feskanich, D., Willett, W., Colditz,G. (2002).Walking and leisure-time activity and risk of hip fracture in postmenopausal women. *Journal of the American Medical Association*, 288, 2300-2306.

[43] Finkelstein, J. S., Brockwell, S. E., Mehta, V., Greendale, G. A., Sowers, M. R., Ettinger, B., Lo, J.C., Johnston, J. M., Cauley, J. A., Danielson, M. E., Neer, R. M. (2008). Bone mineral density changes during the menopause transition in a multiethnic cohort of women. *Journal of Clinical Endocrinology and Metabolism,* 93, 861-868.

[44] Finkelstein, J. S, Lee, M. T., Sowers, M., Ettinger, B., Neer, R. M., Kelsey, J. L., Cauley, J.A., Huang, M., Greendale, G. A. (2002). Ethnic variation in bone density in premenopausal and early perimenopausal women: effects of anthropometric and lifestyle factors. *Journal of Clinical Endocrinology and Metabolism,* 87, 3057-3067.

[45] Fini, M., Salamanna, F., Veronesi, F., Torricelli, P., Nicolini, A., Benedicenti, S., Giavaresi, G. (2012). Role of obesity, alcohol and smoking on bone health. *Front Biosci* (Elite Ed), 4, 2686-2706.

[46] Flynn, M. G., McFarlin, B. K., Phillips, M. D., Stewart, L. K., Timmerman, K. L. (2003). Toll-like receptor 4 and CD14 mRNA expression are lower in resistive exercise-trained elderly women. *Journal of Applied Physiology*, 95(5), 1833-1842.

[47] Food and Nutrition Board, I. o. M., National Academies. Deitary References Intakes (DRIs): Estimated Average Requirements (PDF). Retrieved 10/01/14, from http://www.iom.edu/Activities/Nutrition/ SummaryDRIs/~/media/Files/Activity Files/Nutrition/DRIs/5_Summary Table Tables 1-4.pdf.

[48] Gaffney-Stomberg, E., Insogna, K. L., Rodriguez, N. R., Kerstetter, J. E. (2009). Increasing dietary protein requirements in elderly people for optimal muscle and bone health. *Journal of the American Geriatric Society,* 57 (6), 1073-1079.

[49] Giannopoulou, I., Ploutz-Snyder, L. L., Carhart, R., Weinstock, R. S., Fernhall, B., Goulopoulou, S., & Kanaley, J. A. (2005). Exercise is required for visceral fat loss in postmenopausal women with type 2 diabetes. *Journal of Clinical Endocrinology Metababolism*, 90(3), 1511-1518.

[50] Gómez-Cabello, A., Ara, I., González-Agüero, A., Casajüs, J., Vicente-Rodríguez, G. (2012). Effects of training on bone mass in older adults: a systematic review. *Sports Medicine*, 42(4),301-325.

[51] Gower, B. A., Casazza, K. (2013). Divergent effects of obesity on bone health. *Journal of Clinical Densitometry*, 16(4), 450-454.

[52] Greco, E. A., Fornari, R., Rossi, F., Santiemma, V., Prossomariti, G., Annoscia, C., Migliaccio, S. (2010). Is obesity protective for osteoporosis? Evaluation of bone mineral density in individuals with high body mass index. *International Journal of Clinical Practice*, 64(6), 817-820.

[53] Greiwe, J. S., Cheng, B., Rubin, D. C., Yarasheski, K. E., Semenkovich, C. F. (2001). Resistance exercise decreases skeletal muscle tumor necrosis factor alpha in frail elderly humans. *FASEB J,* 15(2), 475-482.

[54] Guadalupe-Grau, A., Fuentes, T., Guerra, B., Calbet, JAL. (2009). Exercise and bone mass in adults. Sports Medicine, 39(6), 439-468.

[55] Gur, A., Denli, A., Nas, K., Cevik, R., Karakoc, M., Sarac, A.J., Erdogan, F. (2002). Possible pathogenetic role of new cytokines in postmenopausal osteoporosis and changes during calcitonin plus calcium therapy. *Rheumatology International*, 22(5),194-198.

[56] Hannan, M. T., Felson D. T., Anderson J. J. (1992). Bone mineral density in elderly men and women: results from the Framingham osteoporosis study. *Journal of Bone and Mineral Research*, 7, 547-553.

[57] Harrington, M., Cashman, K. D. (2003). High salt intake appears to increase bone resorption in postmenopausal women but high potassium intake ameliorates this adverse effect. *Nutrition Reviews*, 61 (5 Pt 1), 179-183.

[58] Heaney, R. P. (2000). Calcium, dairy products and osteoporosis. *Journal of Nutrition,* 19 (2 Suppl), 83S-99S.

[59] Heaney, R. P., Layman, D. K. (2008). Amount and type of protein influences bone health. *American Journal of Clinical Nutrition*, 87 (5), 1567S-1570S.

[60] Ho-Pham, L. T., Nguyen N. D., Lai, T. Q., Nguyen T. V. (2010). Contributions of lean mass and fat mass to bone mineral density: a study in postmenopausal women. *BMC Musculoskeletal Disorders*, 11, 59-69.

[61] Holt, H.L., Katz, J. N., Reichmann, W. M., Gerlovin, H., Wright, E. A., Hunter, D. J., Jordan, J.M., Keesler, C. L., Losina, E. (2011). Forcasting the burden of advanced knee

osteoarthritis over a 10-year period in a cohort of 60-64 year-old adults. *Osteoarthritis and Cartilage*, 19(1), 44-50.

[62] Hosny, I., Elghawabi, H., Younan, W., Sabbour, A., Gobrial, M. (2012). Beneficial impact of aerobic exercises on bone mineral density in obese premenopausal women under caloric restriction. *Skeletal Radiology*, (4):423-427.

[63] Hsu, Y. H., Venners, S. A., Ierwedow, H. A., Feng, Y., Niu, T., Li, Z., Laird, N., Brain J.D., Cummings, S.R., Bouxsein, M.L. (2006) Relation of body composition, fat mass, and serum lipids to osteoporotic fractures and bone mineral density in Chinese men and women. *American Journal of Clinical Nutrition*, 83, 146-154.

[64] Huang, Q., Gao, B., Wang, L., Hu, Y. Q., Lu, W. G., Yang, L., Liu, J. (2014). Protective effects of myricitrin against osteoporosis via reducing reactive oxygen species and bone-resorbing cytokines. *Toxicology and Applied Pharmacology*, 15, S0041.

[65] Huang, P., Li, S., Shao, M., Qi, Q., Zhao, F., You, J., Liu, Y. (2010). Calorie restriction and endurance exercise share potent anti-inflammatory function in adipose tissues in ameliorating diet-induced obesity and insulin resistance in mice. *Nutritional Metabolism* (London), 7, 59.

[66] Hughes, J. P., McDowell, M. A., Brody, D. J. (2008). Leisure-time physical activity among US adults 60 or more years of age: results from NHANES 1999–2004. *Journal of Physical Activity and Health*, 5(3), 347–355.

[67] Hunter, G. R., Brock, D. W., Byrne, N. M., Chandler-Laney, P. C., Del Corral, P., Gower, B. A. (2010). Exercise training prevents regain of visceral fat for 1 year following weight loss. *Obesity* (Silver Spring), 18(4), 690-695.

[68] Institute of Medicine, F. a. N. B. (2010). Dietary Reference Intakes for Calcium and Vitamin D. Washington, D.C., National Academy Press.

[69] Ishii, S., Cauley, J.A., Greendale, G. A., Danielson, M.E., Nili, N.S., Karlamangla, A. (2012). Ethnic differences in composite indices of femoral neck strength. *Osteoporosis International*, 23, 1381-1390.

[70] Ishii, S., Greendale, J. A., Cauley J. A., Crandall, C. J., Huang, M., Danielson, M. E., Karlamangla, A. S. (2012). Fracture risk assessment without race/ethnicity information. *Journal of Clinical Endocrinology and Metabolism,* 97, 3593-3602.

[71] Itoh, K., Udagawa, N., Kobayashi, K., Suda, K., Li, X., Takami, M., Takahashi, N. (2003). Lipopolysaccharide promotes the survival of osteoclasts via Toll-like receptor 4, but cytokine production of osteoclasts in response to lipopolysaccharide is different from that of macrophages. *Journal of Immunology*, 170(7), 3688-3695.

[72] Jalava, T., Sarna, S., Pylkkanen, L., Mawer, B., Kanis, J.A., Selby, P., Davies, M., Adams, J., Francis, R.M., Robinson, J., McCloskey, E. (2003). Association between vertebral fracture and increased mortality in osteoporotic patients. *Journal of Bone and Mineral Research*, 18, 1254-1260.

[73] Jilka, R. L. (1998). Cytokines, bone remodeling, and estrogen deficiency: a 1998 update. *Bone,* 23(2), 75-81.

[74] Johnell, O, Kanis J. A., Oden A., Johanssen, H., DeLaet C., Delmas, P., Eisman J. A., Fujwara S., Kroger H., Mellstrom, D. (2005). Predictive value of BMD for hip and other fractures. *Journal of Bone and Mineral Research,* 20, 1185-1194.

[75] Jones, G., Nguyen, T., Sambrook, P., Kelly, P.J., Eisman. J.A. (1994). Progressive loss of bone in the femoral neck in elderly people: longitudinal findings from the Dubbo osteoporosis epidemiology study. *British Medical Journal*, 309 (6956), 691-695.

[76] Jung, S. M., Kim, K. W., Yang, C. W., Park, S. H., Ju, J. H. (2014). Cytokine-mediated bone destruction in rheumatoid arthritis. *Journal of Immunology Research*, 10,1155.

[77] Kanis J. A. (2007) A Technical Report: Assessment of osteoporosis at the primary health care level. UK: World Health Organization Collaborating Centre for Metabolic Diseases, University of Sheffield.

[78] Kanis, J. A., Johnell, O., Oden, A., Johansson, H., De Laet, C., Eisman, J. A., Fujiwara, S., Kroger, H., McCloskey, E. V., Mellstrom, D., Melton, L. J.,Pols, H., Reeve, J., Silman, A., Tenenhouse, A. (2005). Smoking and fracture risk: a meta-analysis. *Osteoporosis International*, 16 (2), 155-162.

[79] Kaptoge, S., Welch, A., McTaggart, A., Mulligan, A., Dalzell, N., Day, N.E., Bingham, S., Khaw, K. T., Reeve. J. (2003). Effects of dietary nutrients and food groups on bone loss from the proximal femur in men and women in the 7th and 8th decades of age. *Osteoporosis International,* 14 (5), 418-428.

[80] Kawai, M., dePaula, F. J., Rosen, C. J. (2012). New insights into osteoporosis: the bone-fat connection. *Journal of Internal Medicine*, 272, 317-329.

[81] Kemmler, W., Lauber, D., Weineck, J., Hensen, J., Kalender, W., Engelke, K. (2004). Benefits of 2 years of intense exercise on bone density, physical fitness, and blood lipids in early post-menopausal osteopenic women. *Archives of Internal Medicine*, 164: 1084-1091.

[82] Kerstetter, J. E., O'Brien, K. O., Insogna, K. L. (2003). Dietary protein, calcium metabolism, and skeletal homeostasis revisited. *American Journal of Clinical Nutrition,* 78 (3 Suppl), 584S-592S.

[83] Kerstetter, J. E., O'Brien, K. O., Insogna, K. L. (2003). Low protein intake: the impact on calcium and bone homeostasis in humans. *Journal of Nutrition,* 133 (3), 855S-861S.

[84] Khandewal, S., Chandra, M., Lo, J. C. (2012). Clinical characteristics, bone mineral density and non-vertebral osteoporotic fracture outcomes among post-menopausal US, South Asian women. *Bone*, 51, 1025-1028.

[85] Khera, A., McGuire, D. K., Murphy, S. A., Stanek, H. G., Das, S. R., Vongpatanasin, W., de Lemos, J. A. (2005). Race and gender differences in C-reactive protein levels. *Journal of the American College of Cardiology*, 46(3), 464-469.

[86] Kleerekoper, M., Nelson, D.A., Peterson, E. L., Flynn, M. J., Pawluszka, A.S., Jacobsen, G., Wilson, P. (1994). Reference data for bone mass, calciotropic hormones, and biochemical markers of bone remodeling in older (55-75) postmenopausal white and black women. *Journal of Bone and Mineral Research*, 9, 1267-1276.

[87] Koh, J. M., Khang, Y. H., Jung, C. H., Bae, S., Kim, D. J., Chung, Y. E., Kim, G. S. (2005) Higher circulating hsCRP levels are associated with lower bone mineral density in healthy pre- and postmenopausal women: evidence for a link between systemic inflammation and osteoporosis. *Osteoporosis International,* 16(10),1263–1271.

[88] Kohrt, W. M., Ehsani, A. A., Birge, Jr., S. J, (1997). Effects of exercise involving predominantly either joint-reaction or ground-reaction forces on bone mineral density in older women. *Journal of Bone and Mineral* Research, 12(8), 1253-1261.

[89] Komar, L., Nieves, J., Cosman, F., Rubin, A., Shen, V., Lindsay, R. (1993). Calcium homeostasis of an elderly population upon admission to a nursing home. *Journal of the American Geriatrics Society*, 41 (10), 1057-1064.

[90] Kovacs, C. S. (2005). Calcium and bone metabolism during pregnancy and lactation. *Journal of Mammary Gland Biology and Neoplasia*, 10 (2), 105-118.

[91] Lambert, C. P., Wright, N. R., Finck, B. N., & Villareal, D. T. (2008). Exercise but not diet-induced weight loss decreases skeletal muscle inflammatory gene expression in frail obese elderly persons. *Journal of Applied Physiology*, 105(2), 473-478.

[92] Li, H., Cuartas, E., Cui, W., Choi, Y., Crawford, T. D., Ke, H. Z., Vignery, A. (2005). IL-1 receptor-associated kinase M is a central regulator of osteoclast differentiation and activation. *Journal of Expimental Medicine,* 201(7), 1169-1177.

[93] Liang, M. T. C., Quezada, L., Lau, J. W. Y., Sokmen, B., Spalding, T.W. (2012). Effect of short-term upper-body resistance training on muscular strength, bone metabolic markers, and BMD in premenopausal women. *Journal of Sports Medicine*, 3, 201-208.

[94] Lim, L. S., Harnack, L. J., Lazovich, D., Folsom, A.R. (2004). Vitamin A intake and the risk of hip fracture in postmenopausal women: the Iowa Women's Health Study. *Osteoporosis International*, 15 (7), 552-559.

[95] Lin, P. H., Ginty, F., Appel, L. J., Aickin, M., Bohannon, A., Garnero, P., Barclay, D., Svetkey, L.P. (2003). The DASH diet and sodium reduction improve markers of bone turnover and calcium metabolism in adults. *Journal of Nutrition,* 133 (10), 3130-3136.

[96] Maddalozzo, G. F., Widrick, J. J., Cardinal, B. J., Winters-Stone, K.M., Hoffman, M. A., Snow, C. M. (2007). The effects of hormone replacement therapy and resistance training on spine bone mineral density in early postmenopausal women. *Bone,* 40(5),1244-1251.

[97] McFarlin, B. K., Flynn, M. G., Campbell, W. W., Stewart, L. K., Timmerman, K. L. (2004). TLR4 is lower in resistance-trained older women and related to inflammatory cytokines. *Medicine & Science in Sports & Exercise,* 36(11), 1876-1883.

[98] Meier, D. E., Luckey, M. M., Wallenstein, S., Lapinski, R.H., Catherwood, B. (1992). Racial differences in pre and post menopausal bone homeostasis: association with bone density. *Journal of Bone and Mineral Research,* 7, 1181-1189.

[99] Melton, L. J., Atkinson, E. J., Cooper, C., O'Fallon, W. M., Riggs, B. L. (1999). Vertebral fractures predict subsequent fractures. *Osteoporosis International,* 10, 214-221.

[100] Mullins, N. M., Sinning, W. E. (2005). Effects of resistance training and protein supplementation on bone turnover in young adult women. *Nutrition and Metabolism*, 17(2), 19.

[101] Myers, A. H., Baker, S. P., Van Natta, M. L., Abbey, H., Robinson, E.G. (1991). Risk factors associated with falls and injuries among elderly institutionalized persons. *American Journal of Epidemiology,* 133(11), 1179–1190.

[102] Nagata, M., Kitagawa, J., Miyake, T., Nakahara, Y. (2002). Effects of exercise practice on the maintenance of radius bone mineral density in postmenopausal women. *Journal of Physiological Anthropology and Applied Human Science,* 21(5), 229–234.

[103] National Osteoporosis Foundation. Clinician's Guide to Prevention and Treatment of Osteoporosis, Washington, DC, National Osteoporosis Foundation, 2013.

[104] Nemes, S., Gordon, M., Rogmark, C., Rolfson, O. (2014). Projections of total hip replacement from 2013-2030. *Acta Orthopaedia*, 85(3), 238-243.

[105] Nguyen, N. D., Pongchaiyakul, C., Center J. R., Eisman J. A. & Nguyen T. V. (2005). Identification of high-risk individuals for hip fracture: a 14-year prospective study. *Journal of Bone and Mineral Research*, 20, 1921-1928.

[106] Nguyen T. V., Eisman J. A., Kelly P.J., Sambrook, P.N. (1996). Risk factors for osteoporotic fractures in elderly men. *American Journal of Epidemiology*, 144, 255-263.

[107] Nguyen T. V., Kelly P. J., Sambrook, P. N., Gilbert C., Pocock N. A., Eisman, J. A. (1994). Lifestyle factors and bone density in the elderly: implications for osteoporosis prevention. *Journal of Bone and Mineral Research*, 9, 1339-1346.

[108] Nieves, J. (2005). Osteoporosis: the role of micronutrients. *American Journal of Clinical Nutrition*, 81 (suppl), 1232S-1239s.

[109] Notelovitz, M. (1997). Osteoporosis: prevention, diagnosis and management. Professional Communications., Inc.

[110] Ozturk, Z. A., Yesil, Y., Kuyumcu, M. E., Bilici, M., Ozturk, N., Yesil, N. K., Ariogul, S. (2013). Inverse relationship between neutrophil lymphocyte ratio (NLR) and bone mineral density (BMD) in elderly people. *Archives in Gerontology and Geriatrics*, 57(1), 81-85.

[111] Paalani, M., Lee, J. W., Haddad, E., Tonstad, S. (2011). Determinants of inflammatory markers in a bi-ethnic population. *Ethnic Diseases*, 21(2), 142-149.

[112] Palombaro, K. (2005). Effects of walking-only interventions on bone mineral density at various skeletal sites, a meta-analysis. *Journal of Geriatric Physical Therapy*, 28,102-107.

[113] Pan, W., Borovac, J., Spicer, Z., Hoenderop, J. G., Bindels, R. J., Shull, G. E., Doschak, M. R., Cordat, E., Alexander, R. T. (2012). The epithelial sodium/proton exchanger, NHE3, is necessary for renal and intestinal calcium (re)absorption. *Renal Physiology-American Journal of Physiology,* 302 (8), F943-956.

[114] Patsch, J. M., Li, X., Baum, T., Yap, S. P., Karampinos, D.C., Schwartz, A. V., Link, T. M. (2013). Bone marrow fat composition as a novel imaging biomarker in postmenopausal women with prevalent fragility fractures. *Journal of Bone and Mineral Research*, 28, 1721-1728.

[115] Phillips, M. D., Flynn, M. G., McFarlin, B. K., Stewart, L. K., Timmerman, K. L., Ji, H. (2008). Resistive exercise blunts LPS-stimulated TNF-alpha and Il-1 beta. *International Journal of Sports Medicine,* 29(2), 102-109.

[116] Poole, K. E., Treece, G. M., Gee, A. H., Brown, J. P., McClung, M. R., Wang, A., Libanati, C. (2014). Denosumab Rapidly Increases Cortical Bone in Key Locations of the Femur: A 3D Bone Mapping Study in Women with Osteoporosis. *Journal of Bone and Mineral Research.* 4 (Epub ahead of print).

[117] Putnam M. S., Wu, E. W., Lee, H., Neer R. M., Schindler E., Taylor, A. P., Cheston, E., Bouxsein M. L., Finkelstein, J. S. (2013). Differences in skeletal microstructure and strength in African-American and white women. *Journal of Bone and Mineral Research*, 28, 2177-2185.

[118] Reid, I. R. (2002). Relationships among body mass, its components and bone. Bone, 31, 547-555.

[119] Reid, I. R., Evans, M. C., Ames R.W. (1994). Volumetric bone density of the lumbar spine is related to fat mass but not lean mass in normal postmenopausal women. *Osteoporosis International*, 4, 362-367.

[120] Ricci, T. A., Heymsfield, S. B., Pierson, R. N., Stahl, T., Chowdhury, H. A., Shapses, S.A. (2001). Moderate energy restriction increases bone resorption in obese postmenopausal women. *American Journal of Clinical Nutrition,* 73(2),347–352.

[121] Riedt, C. S., Cifuentes, M., Stahl, T., Chowdhury, H.A., Schlussel, Y., Shapses, S.A. (2005). Overweight postmenopausal women lose bone with moderate weight reduction and 1 g/day calcium intake. *Journal of Bone and Mineral Research* 20(3),455–463.

[122] Riggs, B. L., Melton, L. J. (1992). The prevention and treatment of osteoporosis. *New England Journal of Medicine*, 327, 620-627.

[123] Ross, P. D., Norimatsu, H., Davis, J. W., Yano, K., Wasnich, R.D., Fujiwara, S., Hosoda, Y., Melton, L. J. (1991). A comparison of hip fracture incidence among native Japanese, Japanese Americans, Mexicans, and Caucasians. *American Journal of Epidemiology*, 133, 801-809.

[124] Ryan, A. S., Treuth, M. S., Hunter, G. R., Elahi, D. (1998). Resistive training maintains bone mineral density in post-menopausal women. *Calcified Tissue International,* 62, 295–299.

[125] Russell-Aulet, M., Wang, J., Thornton, J.C., Colt, E.W.D., Pierson, R.N. (1993). Bone mineral density and mass in a cross-sectional study of white and Asian women. *Journal of Bone and Mineral Research*, 8, 575-582.

[126] Santaliestra-Pasias, A. M., Mouratidou, T., Verbestel, V., Bammann, K., Molnar, D., Sieri, S., Veidebaum, T., Marild, S., Lissner, L., Hadjigeorgiou, C., Reisch, L., DeBourdeaudhuij, I., Moreno, L.A. (2013). Physical activity and sedentary behavior in European children:the IDEFICS study. *Public Health and Nutrition*, 8, 1-12.

[127] Schett, G., Kiechl, S., Weger, S., Pederiva, A., Mayr, A., Petrangeli, M., Willeit, J. (2006). High-sensitivity C-reactive protein and risk of nontraumatic fractures in the Bruneck study. *Archives of Internal Medicine*, 166(22), 2495-2501.

[128] Scheidt-Nave, C., Bismar, H., Leidig-Bruckner, G., Woitge, H., Seibel, M.J., Ziegler, R., Pfeilschifter, J. (2001). Serum interleukin 6 is a major predictor of bone loss in women specific to the first decade past menopause. *Journal of Clinical Endocrinology and Metabolism*, 86(5),2032–2042.

[129] Selvin, E., Halushka, M. K., Rawlings, A. M., Hoogeveen, R. C., Ballantyne, C. M., Coresh, J., Astor, B. C. (2013). sRAGE and risk of diabetes, cardiovascular disease, and death. *Diabetes,* 62(6), 2116-2121.

[130] Silva, H. G., Mendonca, L. M., Conceicao, F. L., Zahar, S. E., & Farias, M. L. (2007). Influence of obesity on bone density in postmenopausal women. *Arquivos Brasilerios Endocrinologia e Metabologia*, 51(6), 943-949.

[131] Silverman, N., Nicklas, B., Ryan, A. (2009). Addition of aerobic exercise to a weight loss program increases BMD, with an associated reduction in inflammation in overweight postmenopausal women. *Calcified Tissue International*, 84(4), 257-265.

[132] Slentz, C. A., Aiken, L. B., Houmard, J. A., Bales, C. W., Johnson, J. L., Tanner, C. J., Kraus, W. E. (2005). Inactivity, exercise, and visceral fat. STRRIDE: a randomized, controlled study of exercise intensity and amount. *Journal of Applied Physiology*, 99(4), 1613-1618.

[133] Stewart, L. K., Flynn, M. G., Campbell, W. W., Craig, B. A., Robinson, J. P., Timmerman, K. L., Talbert, E. (2007). The influence of exercise training on inflammatory cytokines and C-reactive protein. *Medicine and Science in Sports and Exercise,* 39(10), 1714-1719.

[134] Strengel, S. V., Kemmler, W., Pintag, R., Beeskow, C., Weineck, J., Lauber, D., Kalender, W. A., Engelke, K. (2005). Power Training is More Effective than Strength Training for Maintaining Bone Mineral Density in Postmenopausal Women. *Journal of Applied Physiology*, 99(1), 181-188.

[135] Sternfeld, B., Dugan, S. (2012). Physical Activity and Health During the Menopausal Transition. *Obstentrics and Gynecology Clinics of North America,* 38(3), 537-566.

[136] Taafee, D. R., Snow-Harter, C., Connolly, D.A., Robinson, T.L., Brown, M.D.,

[137] Marcus, R. (1995). Differential effects of swimming versus weightbearing activity on bone mineral status of eumenorrheic athletes. *Journal of Bone and Mineral Researc*h, 10, 586–593.

[138] Tanumihardo, S.A. (2013). Vitamin A and bone health: the balancing act. *Journal of Clinical Densitometry*, 16(4), 414-419.

[139] Taylor, R. S., Ashton, K. E., Moxham, T., Hooper, L., Ebrahim, S. (2011). Reduced dietary salt for the prevention of cardiovascular disease: a meta-analysis of randomized trials. *American Journal of Hypertension,* 24(8), 843-853.

[140] Telford, R. M., Telford, R. D., Cunningham, R. B., Cochrane, T., Davey, R., Waddington, G. (2013). Longitudinal patterns of physical activity in children aged 8 to 12 years: the LOOK study. *International Journal of Behavioral Nutrition, and Physical Acti*vity, 10, 1-12.

[141] Tenta, R., Moschonis, G., Koutsilieris, M., Manios, Y. (2011). Calcium and vitamin D supplementation through fortified dairy products counterbalances seasonal variations of bone metabolism indices: the Postmenopausal Health Study. *European Journal of Nutrition*, 50 (5), 341-349.

[142] Thomas, E. L., Brynes, A. E., McCarthy, J., Goldstone, A. P., Hajnal, J. V., Saeed, N., Bell, J. D. (2000). Preferential loss of visceral fat following aerobic exercise, measured by magnetic resonance imaging. *Lipids,* 35(7), 769-776.

[143] Timmen, M., Hidding, H., Wieskotter, B., Baum, W., Pap, T., Raschke, M. J., Stange, R. (2014). Influence of antiTNF-alpha antibody treatment on fracture healing under chronic inflammation. *BMC Musculoskeletal Disorders,* 15, 184.

[144] Timmerman, K. L., Flynn, M. G., Coen, P. M., Markofski, M. M., Pence, B. D. (2008). Exercise training-induced lowering of inflammatory (CD14+CD16+) monocytes: a role in the anti-inflammatory influence of exercise? *Journal of Leukocyte Biology*, 84(5), 1271-1278.

[145] U.S. Department of Agriculture, A. R. S., Beltsville Research Center, Food Surveys Research Group What we eat in American, NHANES 2005-2006: Usual Nutrient intakes from food and water compated to 1997 dietary reference intakes for Vitamin D, Calcium, Phospohrous, and Magnesium.

[146] Valimaki, V. V., Alfthan, H., Lehmuskallio, E., Loyttyniemi, E., Sahi, T., Stenman, U.H., Suominen, H., Valimaki, M.J. (2004). Vitamin D status as a determinant of peak bone mass in young Finnish men. *Journal of Clinical Endocrinology and Metabolism*, 89 (1), 76-80.

[147] Vásquez, E., Benjamin, S.A., Lenore, G., Daniel, O., Leonor, C. (2013). Racial and ethnic differences in physical activity and bone density: *National Health and Nutrition Examination Survey*, 2007–2008. Preventing Chronic Disease, 10, 1-10.

[148] Verbruggen, A., De Clerck, L. S., Bridts, C. H., Van Offel, J. F., Stevens, W. J. (1999). Flow cytometrical determination of interleukin 1beta, interleukin 6 and tumour necrosis

factor alpha in monocytes of rheumatoid arthritis patients; relation with parameters of osteoporosis. *Cytokine,* 11(11), 869-874.

[149] Walker, M. D., Babbar, R., Opotowsky, A., McMahon, D. J., Liu, G., Bilezikan, J. P. (2007). Determinants of bone mineral density in Chinese-American women. *Osteoporosis International*, 18, 471-478.

[150] Walker, M.D., Novotny, R., Bilezikian, J.P., Weaver, C.M. (2008). Race and Diet Interactions in the Acquisition, Maintenance and Loss of Bone. *Journal of Nutrition,* 138(6), 1256S-1260S.

[151] Walston, J. D., Fallin, M. D., Cushman, M., Lange, L., Psaty, B., Jenny, N., Reiner, A. (2007). IL-6 gene variation is associated with IL-6 and C-reactive protein levels but not cardiovascular outcomes in the Cardiovascular Health Study. *Human Genetics*, 122(5), 485-494.

[152] Wang, M. C., Bachrach L. K., Van Loan, M., Hudes, M., Flegal, K. M., Crawford, P. B. (2005). The relative contributions of lean tissue mass and fat mass to bone density in young woman. *Bone*, 37, 474-481.

[153] Wang, X. F., Duan, Y., Beck, T. J., Seeman, E. (2005). Varying contributions of growth and ageing to racial and sex differences in femoral neck structure and strength in old age. *Bone,* 36, 978-986.

[154] Warren, M., Petit, M.A., Hannan, P. J., Schmitz, K.H. (2008). Strength training effects on bone mineral density in premenopausal women. *Medicine and Science in Sports and Exercise,* 40(7), 1282-1288.

[155] Waugh, E. J., Lam, M.A., Hawker, G. A., McGowan, J., Papainnou, A., Cheung, A. M., Hodsman, A. B., Leslie, W. D., Siminoski, K., Jamal, S.A. (2009). Risk factors for low bone mass in healthy 40-60 year old women: a systematic review of the literature. *Osteoporosis International*, 20, 1-21.

[156] Weber, P. (1999). The role of vitamins in the prevention of osteoporosis--a brief status report. *International Journal for Vitamin and Nutrition Research,* 69 (3), 194-197.

[157] Weisman, S. M. (2005). The calcium connection to bone health across a woman's lifespan: a roundtable. *Journal of Reproductive Medicine*, 50 (11 Suppl), 879-884.

[158] Whelton, S. P., Narla, V., Blaha, M. J., Nasir, K., Blumenthal, R. S., Jenny, N. S., Michos, E. D. (2014). Association between resting heart rate and inflammatory biomarkers (high-sensitivity C-reactive protein, interleukin-6, and fibrinogen) (from the Multi-Ethnic Study of Atherosclerosis). *American Journal of Cardiology,* 113(4), 644-649.

[159] Wilkin, L. D., Jackson, M. C., Sims, T. D., Haddock, B. L. (2010). Racial/ethnic differences in bone mineral density of young adults. *International Journal of Exercise Science*, 3, 197-205.

[160] Winters, K., Snow, C. (2000). Detraining reverses positive effects of exercise on the musculoskeletal system in premenopausal women. *Journal of Bone and Mineral Research*, 15(12):2495-2503.

[161] Winters-Stone, K. M., Snow, C. M. (2006). Site specific response of bone to exercise in premenopausal women. *Bone,* 39(6),1203-1209.

[162] WHO (2003). Prevention and management of osteoporosis. Report of a WHO study group, World Health Organization, Geneva. Technical report series 919, 1-165.

[163] Wong, P. K., Christie, J. J., Wark, J. D. (2007). The effects of smoking on bone health. *Clinical Science*, 113 (5), 233-241.

[164] Wu, Q., Lefante, J. J., Rice, J. C., Magnus, J. H. (2011). Age, race, weight, and gender impact normative values of bone mineral density. *Gender Medicine*, 8, 189-201.

[165] Yamagishi, S., Matsui, T. (2010). Advanced glycation end products, oxidative stress and diabetic nephropathy. *Oxidative Medicine and Cell Longevity*, 3(2), 101-108.

[166] Yasuda, H. (2013). Anti-RANKL antibody was approved for the treatment of osteoporosis in Japan. Nihon Rinsho Meneki *Gakkai Kaishi,* 36(4), 209-216.

[167] Yilmaz, H., Uyfun, M., Yilmaz, T. S., Namuslu, M., Inan, O., Taskin, A., Kosar, A. (2014). Neutrophil-lymphocyte ratio may be superior to C-reactive protein for predicting the occurrence of postmenopausal osteoporosis. *Endocrinology Regulation*, 48(1), 25-33.

[168] Zehnacker, C. H., Bemis-Dougherty, A. (2007). Effects of weighted exercises on bone mineral density in post menopausal women: a systematic review. *Journal of Geriatric Physical Therapy*, 30 (2), 79-88.

[169] Zheng, S. X., Vrindts, Y., Lopez, M., De Groote, D., Zangerle, P. F., Collette, J., Reginster, J. Y. (1997). Increase in cytokine production (IL-1 beta, IL-6, TNF-alpha but not IFN-gamma, GM-CSF or LIF) by stimulated whole blood cells in postmenopausal osteoporosis. *Maturitas,* 26(1), 63-71.

In: Bone Disorders, Screening and Treatment
Editor: Aubrey M. Stone

ISBN: 978-1-63482-155-1


*Chapter 2*

# Pregnancy and Bone Mineral Density Changes

***William W. K. To**[*1] and Margaret W. N. Wong[2]*
[1]MD, FRCOG, FHKAM (Obs/Gyn), Chief-of-Service and Consultant Obstetrician, Department of Obstetrics & Gynaecology United Christian Hospital, Hong Kong
[2]MD, FRCS (Edin), FHKAM (Orthopaedic Surgery)
Honorary Professor, Department of Orthopaedics and Traumatology
The Chinese University of Hong Kong, Hong Kong

## Abstract

Recent research has shown that pregnancy could be associated be bone mineral density (BMD) loss. The patterns of BMD changes in pregnancy have been evaluated in many recent studies. This BMD loss during the course of pregnancy is largely transient, and should recover within a relatively short period of time in the postpartum period. However, this pregnancy related BMD loss can also become chronic if postpartum recovery fail to occur or was not complete, giving rise to increased risks of osteoporosis in later pre- and post-menopausal life. While radiological methods have been used in the past for monitoring such BMD changes, recent research have shown that the use of quantitative ultrasound for the monitoring of BMD changes in pregnancy is feasible, and is particularly advantageous as it is free from radiation side effects as compared to other standard radiological techniques for BMD measurements, such as dual energy X-ray absorptiometry or quantitative tomography. The use of quantitative USG measurements on different bony sites, including the os calcis or phalanges during pregnancy has been reported and compared. The use of serial quantitative USG has allowed more detailed research into such pregnancy related BMD changes, and significant factors that will influence this change, such as body weight, body fat composition, parity or other antenatal obstetric conditions have been evaluated. Pregnancy symptoms such as low back pain have been associated with BMD changes during pregnancy, while active

[*] Corresponding author: William WK To: Email: towkw@ha.org.hk

exercises on the physiological BMD changes during pregnancy have shown that the BMD loss was apparently less compared to those that were not regularly exercising.

Epidemiological data have shown that parity and lactation do not have significant detrimental effects on bone health in later life. This is consistent with the observation that BMD loss during pregnancy and lactation usually recovers within a few years. Overall, pregnancy appears to be a protective or neutral factor against menopausal fractures. The key findings of the current studies would be summarized in this chapter.

# 1. Introduction

Normal adaptative responses during pregnancy and lactation allow for adequate delivery of minerals to the fetus or infant, while at the same time protecting to a certain degree the maternal skeleton. The maternal skeleton remains the most important source of calcium to the fetus during pregnancy [1]. Theoretically, bone mass may decrease in response to this transfer of calcium from the maternal skeleton, bone mineral density may also increase as a result of the rise in oestrogen levels in late pregnancy, so that overall bone mineral density may decrease, remain unchanged or increase [2]. The full term neonate contains around 30 g calcium in it skeleton while the maternal skeleton, on the other hand, should contain around 1000 g of calcium [3]. Thus, a theoretical magnitude of bone loss of 3-4 % is logical under the assumption that the fetal calcium requirement is completely supplied by the maternal skeleton. This calculation, however, has not taken into account the maternal calcium homeostasis and adaptation of this homeostasis during pregnancy [4]. However, it is obvious that pregnancy and lactation do pose significant stress to maternal calcium metabolism. The long term consequences of pregnancy and lactation to bone health and possible association with subsequent osteoporosis in menopausal age have also been studied, but the results continued to be controversial.

# 2. Physiology of Calcium Metabolism in Pregnancy

Pregnancy has been classically called a ‘physiologic absorptive hypercalciuric state” [5]. The increase in intestinal absorption might reflect an elevation in circulating 1,25-dihydroxyvitamin D (calcitriol) or possibly a direct intestinal effect of oestrogen to stimulate calcium transport Increases in calcitriol concentrations from 15 – 60pg/ml in the non-pregnant state to 80-120 pg/ml in the pregnant state. The process might begin as early as the first trimester, and be achieved in late pregnancy [6]. Calcitriol is produced in the placenta as well as in the kidneys in pregnancy. Though the circulating vitamin D binding protein increases, ‘free’ calcitriol concentrations are also elevated, as are circulating albumin-adjusted calcium or ionised calcium concentrations and urinary calcium excretion [7]. While the calcium balance in pregnant women is positively maintained by these mechanisms, there is no consistent relationship found between intestinal calcium absorption and either dietary calcium intake or any index of calcitriol “bioavailability” in pregnant women. In contrast, although maternal calcitriol production increases with lactation, it does not achieve the same concentrations seen during pregnancy, and there is no associated increase in intestinal calcium absorption [6]. Instead, calcium is conserved by a renal mechanism, with decreased urinary calcium excretion with lactation that may remain low for as long as six months post-weaning. Under normal circumstances, the greater efficiency of intestinal calcium absorption during pregnancy meets the calcium demand. An interesting classical study on bone architecture compared transilial bone biopsy samples from two groups of pregnant women in first trimester and third trimester of pregnancy. It was shown that there was a fluctuation in the cancellous bone volume in which early temporary bone loss through trabecular thinning is restored entirely through the addition of new trabeculae to produce a complex system of thinner but more numerous bars near term [8]. How such changes in bone architecture should be interpreted in terms of bone density changes as measured by various techniques remained uncertain. There is at present no consensus as to the impact of reproductive events on bone mineral density on the ultimate BMD after pregnancy or in later life. The results from observational studies available in the literature are conflicting and controversial.

## 3. Studies Using Radiological Methods to Monitor BMD Changes in Pregnancy

Various earlier longitudinal studies have utilized radiological methods such as single-photon absorptiometry (SPA) and dual energy X-ray absorptiometry (DXA), which are usually regarded as inadvisable or contraindicated during pregnancy because of risks of radiation exposure (Table 1).

Thus, the ways to get around this risk during pregnancy would be to scan the woman before conception and then in the early postpartum period after her pregnancy. The need to recruit subjects prospectively even before they are pregnant posed to be difficult and often unfeasible. The sample size of such studies is often limited, as the source of patients that potentially could be recruited into such studies would also be limited. In addition, no direct measurements of BMD could be made during the course of pregnancy itself.

### 3.1. Studies Showing no BMD Loss in Pregnancy

Using single photon absorptiometry to measure forearm BMD in thirteen women, Christiansen [9] showed that the values remained constant, and concluded that total body calcium is constant during pregnancy. Sowers [10] measured femoral BMD using dual photon densitometry in 32 women before conception and within 2 weeks after delivery and compared these with a group of non-pregnant controls. No significant mean BMD loss was observed. In addition, smaller body size pregnant women were likely to have femoral BMD increases during pregnancy than the controls. It was concluded that fetal demand for calcium has a minimal effect on BMD at parturition and smaller women may experience a slight increase in femoral BMD compared with controls. Another study measured BMD of the distal radius of the forearm using dual energy X-ray absorptiometry (DXA) in 22 pregnant women in a longitudinal fashion, and found that in none of the women were there any noticeable changes

**Table 1. Precision and radiation dose of currently used techniques for the assessment of bone density (modified from Jergas [64])**

| Technique | Accuracy (%) | Precision (%) | Radiation exposure (uSv) |
|---|---|---|---|
| Conventional radiography | | | |
| Lateral thoracic spine | -- | -- | 500-1100 |
| Lateral lumbar spine | -- | -- | 1300-2700 |
| Photodensitometry (hand) | 5 | 1-2 | < 5 |
| Single photon absorptiometry/ Single X- ray absorptiometry | 1-2 | 4-6 | 1 |
| Dual photon absorptiometry | | | |
| Lumbar spine PA pencil beam | 1-10 | 1 | 1-2.5 |
| Lumbar spine PA fan beam | | | 10-60 |
| Lumbar spine lateral | 8-10 | 1-6 | 3 |
| Proximal femur | 6 | 1-2 | 1-6 |
| Radius | 5 | 1 | 1 |
| Whole body | 3 | 1 | 3 |
| Quantitative computerized tomography | | | |
| Singe energy QCT | 5-15 | 1.5 -4 | 50-300 |
| Dual energy QCT | 3-6 | 4-6 | 150-1000 |
| Peripheral quantitative computerized | | | |
| tomography | 2-8 | 1-2 | 1 |
| Radius trabecular | 2-8 | 1-2 | 1 |
| Radius total | | | |
| Quantitative Ultrasound | | | |
| Os Calcis | 3-5 | 3-6 | Nil |

in BMD during pregnancy. No significant change in BMD occurred during the 12 month postpartum period in the 11 non-lactating women, while the rest that breast fed had significant drop in BMD at 1, 3, 6 months and 12 months postpartum. The findings supported BMD loss with lactation but not during pregnancy [11]. Moreover, in a review of such radiological methods by Sowers [2], longitudinal studies using the more crude single or dual-photon absorptiometry were inconsistent and either showed no change or a loss of femoral neck and mid-radius BMD.

### 3.2. Studies Showing Significant BMD Loss

Other studies, however, have shown opposite results. In a small sample of six healthy active pregnant women, Drinkwater [12] measured BMD at 7 sites using single and dual photon absorptiometry and compared with 25 non-pregnant controls. BMD was found to decrease significantly in the femoral neck and radial shaft but increased in the tibial shaft. A 3.3% decrease in the lumbar spine BMD was also observed, which returned to pre-pregnant levels at the postpartum period during lactation. Bone loss at the femoral neck continued during lactation.

Similarly, in a prospective study of 38 Hungarian women in their first full term pregnancy [13], BMD measurements were made at the lumbar spine (L2-L4) and forearm (distal 33%) and ultradistal region of the radius before conception, after delivery, and at 6 and 12 months postpartum. The patients were grouped according to the duration of lactation. There was a significant decrease in BMD between baseline pre-conception and delivery in the lumbar spine, ultra-distal radius and forearm. The authors concluded that calcium needed for fetal skeletal growth during pregnancy was gained from maternal trabecular and cortical sites, which were not adequately compensated for by maternal adaptations. The calcium needed for infant growth during lactation was drawn mainly from maternal trabecular bone, as reflected by the persistent fall in BMD in the lumbar spine but not the radius. The effect of pregnancy and lactation on the maternal bone mass was spontaneously compensated for after weaning.

In another study, Kaur [14] was able to recruit a substantial number of normal young women who were contemplating pregnancy and BMD was measured pre-conceptually using standard DXA equipment. Those who subsequently became pregnant were measured again soon after delivery and at several time points in the postpartum year. Out of 122 recruits, 42 were pregnant during the study period and these were compared with 30 women who failed to conceive within the 24 months of the study. The mean time to follow up in the pregnant group was 14 months (SD $\pm$ 3) and the mean time to follow up for the controls was 16 months (SD $\pm$ 3). There was no difference in the baseline BMD of the pregnant and the control groups, nor was there any correlation between pre-conceptual BMD at the various sites and dietary calcium intake. In the patients who became pregnant, there was a small but statistically insignificant decrease in BMD at all the measured sites (lumbar spine, total hip, trochanter and femoral neck) at the post-delivery assessment. The total number of women with a decrease in BMD in excess of the least significant change (LSC) at any site was 20 (47.6%), while only 2 women showed a gain in BMD that exceeded the LSC at the spine and hip. There was no correlation between the change in BMD during pregnancy and the pre-conceptual value at any site. On the other hand, there was a slight increase in BMD at all measurement sites in those who failed to become pregnant, with a small number of women showing gains greater than the least significant changes and none with decrease in BMD greater than the least significant changes. One remarkable point of this study is the inclusion of a non-pregnant control group. Very few studies of this nature have included a control group, but this does provide some assessment of drift in the densitometric technique and controls for age- related changes in BMD as well as other clinical characteristics. Although the loss of BMD during pregnancy was relatively small and not statistically significant, 40.5% of the women in this cohort showed a fall in BMD of more than 5% at the trochanteric region, indicating that for a significant proportion of women, the loss of BMD at specific sites was significant. The pattern of BMD loss described in this study was in contrast to the concept that pregnancy-associated osteoporosis involves the spine more commonly than the hip [15].

### 3.3. Differential Bone Loss at Different Bone Sites

Differential changes in BMD in different bone sites have also been found in different studies. In a study by Naylor [16], BMD increased in the arms (+2.8%) and legs (1.9%) but decreased in the pelvis (-3.2%) and lumbar spine (-4.6%), a phenomenon that was described as redistribution of bone mineral, consistent with the hypothesis that decrease in bone mass during pregnancy occurred more at trabecular bone sites, while sites consisting of cortical bone showed either no change or even a tendency towards gains in BMD. In an older study, Lamke [17] found a similar pattern with loss of trabecular bone structure and gain of cortical bone at different sites, or even within the same distal forearm bone. In a more recent prospective study with 34 women with normal pregnancies, cortical and trabecular bone BMD were measured in the first and third trimesters using peripheral quantitative computerized tomography (QCT) in conjunction with a panel of bone metabolism parameters. It was found that cortical bone density was unaffected by pregnancy while trabecular bone density changes showed wide individual variations, ranging from +1.3 to -20.7% per year, which were identified as fast losers and slow losers by the investigators. Serum osteocalcin levels were lower in slow versus fast bone losers in both trimesters [18].

Several explanations could be offered for the conflicting results. Most of the data consists of cross-sectional surveys instead of large-scale longitudinal measurements through one or several complete reproductive cycles, and often involves small number of women. The BMD measurements studied also involved various bone sites measured by various methods. Conflicting results also arises when within the same set of data, some bone sites showed decrease in BMD, while other sites showed no decline or even overcompensation. In addition, both technological and methodological issues contribute to this uncertainty. Different studies have used different radiological techniques to measure BMD changes, and each of these methods would have their specific coefficients of variation and sensitivity in documenting the changes. The time points where such BMD measurements were made are also very variable. As many of these studies involved radiological methods of measurement, which are relatively contraindicated in pregnancy, the measurements were often arranged to be done some time before conception/ pregnancy, and then after pregnancy and delivery or in the post-weaning state, rather than directly monitoring BMD during the course of pregnancy. The different time points in measurement will need to be taken into account when interpreting such results.

## 4. Calcium Supplementation Affecting BMD Changes in Pregnancy

The role calcium supplementation has been a controversial issue. So far, few studies have directly examined the effects of calcium supplementation on BMD in pregnancy. In a small randomized control trial on Chinese pregnant women, subjects were assigned to usual diet, usual diet + milk powder supplemented with 35 mg calcium/day, or usual diet + milk powder + oral calcium supplements 600mg/day. Postpartum DXA showed a dose dependent relationship between calcium intake and BMD. The total body and spine BMD values were significantly higher in subjects with calcium and milk supplementation than controls. Significant decreases in changes in urinary hydroxyproline and significant increases in serum osteocalcin were seen in the calcium/ milk supplemented groups than in the controls. The authors suggested that calcium and milk supplementation during pregnancy is associated with higher postnatal BMD values and might suppress bone resorption in Chinese women with habitual low calcium diets [19].

In a study on 34 British women, DXA was performed before conception and within 2 weeks after conception, and the data was compared to non-pregnant controls and correlated with their calcium intake during pregnancy. The pregnancy group experienced significant decreases in total bone mineral content (BMC), areal BMD, and bone area adjusted BMC at the spine, and total hip by 1-4 %. Weight change was a positive predictor of skeletal change at the spine, hip and radius, but calcium intake was not a significant predictor of skeletal change in either pregnant or non-pregnant women. It was concluded that calcium intake was not a significant predictor of skeletal response to pregnancy in well –nourished women [20]. Thus, it could be seen that the effects of calcium intake on BMD changes during pregnancy are likely to be variable and dependent on the baseline nutritional state of the woman.

## 5. Pathological Osteoporosis Associated with Pregnancy

While the studies quoted in the previous section have described bone loss during and after pregnancy, such loss should be physiological and mild. The risks of sustaining fractures during pregnancy due to such degree of BMD should indeed be rare, as these women are still in reproductive age groups and should still have a sufficiently high level of bone mass to prevent against atraumatic fractures [21]. However, rarely, fractures are sustained during pregnancy in those with transient but severe loss of bone mass during their gestational period. This should be considered as a pathological process, commonly named transient osteoporosis of pregnancy.

Transient osteoporosis of pregnancy is a rare, idiopathic, self limiting condition typically occurring in the third trimester of pregnancy. The mean gestation to occur is usually reported to be around 33 weeks, but can range from 6 weeks to term [22]. It almost always affects a single hip although bilateral presentation or knee involvement [23] and lumbar spine involvement have also been reported [22].

Transient osteoporosis in pregnancy occurring in the hip usually presents with a sudden, severe onset of unilateral groin pain with no history or trauma. The patient may be unable to bear weight, and pain is elicited by hip rotation, but a full range of movement is often possible [24]. X-ray examination should be avoided in pregnancy, but magnetic resonance imaging should reveal mottled low signal intensity of bone marrow on T1 weighted images, and high signal on T2 weighted images suggestive of bone marrow oedema [22].

Hip fractures secondary to transient osteoporosis of pregnancy may occur in up to 15% of cases, but such fractures can occasionally be bilateral [25]. The process should be self limiting and symptoms should thus resolve within 3 to 6 months after delivery. However, additional treatment for enhancing BMD has also been attempted, such as treatment with vitamin D, calcitriol and alendronate or risedronic acid for up to 2 years until BMD increased to reasonable levels [26].

The aetiology of transient osteoporosis remains unclear, and proposed mechanisms included mechanical compression of the obturator nerve, reflex sympathetic dystrophy, disturbance of hormonal return, hormonal factors, transient synovitis or an early phase of avascular necrosis, though none could be proven [22]. The diagnosis of transient osteoporosis of pregnancy should be suspected when hip pain occurs during pregnancy or in the postpartum period, as it may lead to acetabular or femoral neck fractures, but should be considered as a pathological condition of entirely different in aetiology to the physiological BMD changes observed in normal pregnancies.

## 6. The Use of Quantitative USG for Monitoring BMD Changes in Pregnancy

Quantitative ultrasonography (QUS) offers an inexpensive, radiation-free method by which to assess BMD and bone quality during pregnancy. The use of such methods allows recruitment of subjects from a general low risk obstetric clinic that would have characteristics similar to the general obstetric population. Larger sample sizes could be achieved as the measurements are simple and non-invasive. Despite such advantages, the use of QUS for monitoring BMD changes in pregnancy and after delivery has often been challenged because of the lower precision of such techniques with a larger coefficient of variation, thus limiting the least minimal change that can be measurable by such systems (Table 1). In addition, QUS measurement parameters often could not be directly correlated to radiological BMD data, which are regarded as the gold standard.

The current studies that utilized quantitative ultrasound to survey BMD changes in pregnancy basically used either calcaneal/ os calcis or phalangeal measurements. The major difference in the use of these two different sites is that calcaneal ultrasound would measure speed of sound (SOS) as well as broadband ultrasound attenuation (BUA) and then yield either a stiffness value or simulated BMD value; phalangeal ultrasound would yield amplitude adjusted SOS and bone transmission time values. The calcaneous anatomically consists of cancellous or trabecular bone, whereas the phalanges consist largely of cortical bone. Thus, it is expected that the magnitude of changes in bone density parameters during pregnancy would be larger in the calcaneous as compared to the phalanges. The coefficient of variation for SOS and BUA parameters from calcaneal measurements are theoretically larger than the SOS and bone transmission time measurements from phalangeal ultrasound. However, as the magnitude of change in the former are also larger, the changes observed should still be higher than the least significant change that could be measured based on the given coefficient of variation. Some QUS systems, such as the Hologic Sahara machine, can give a simulated BMD value as estimated from the SOS and BUA values [Figure 1].

There are also system specific reference ranges for these simulated BMD values in accordance with different age groups [Table 2]. However, given the small sample size in many of the studies published in the literature, there is indeed room to argue about the genuine validity of the differences in the ultrasound parameters that were detected, so that one would question whether such findings were “real or imaginary” [27]. Therefore, in order to override such random error, large sample sizes are mandatory in such studies.

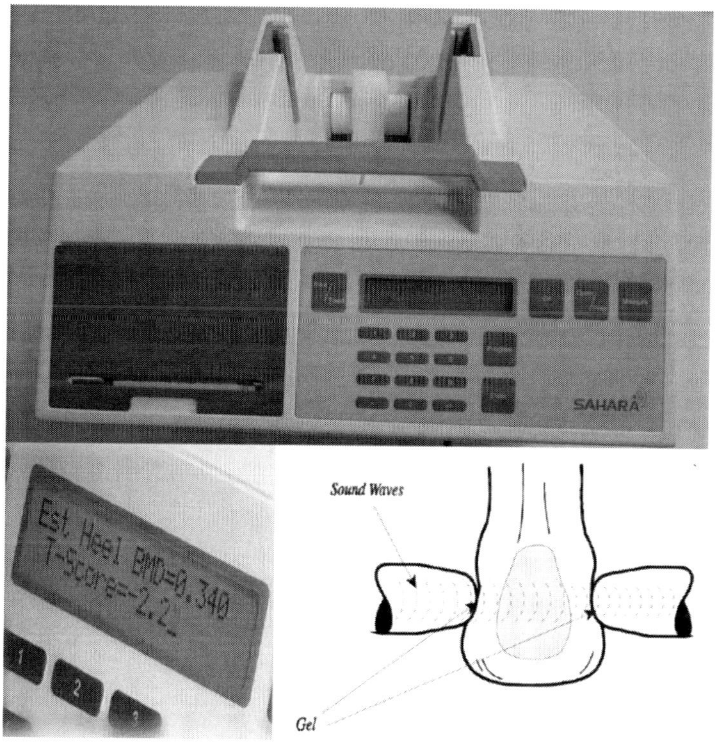


Figure 1. Hologic Sahara Clinical Bone Sonometer quantitative ultrasound system.

**Table 2. Hologic Sahara system estimated os calcis BMD values versus age**

| Age (years) | Estimated os calcis BMD ( g/cm$^2$) | Standard Deviation ( g/cm$^2$) |
|---|---|---|
| 25 | 0.581 | 0.112 |
| 35 | 0.555 | 0.112 |
| 45 | 0.562 | 0.112 |
| 55 | 0.545 | 0.112 |
| 65 | 0.471 | 0.112 |
| 75 | 0.436 | 0.112 |
| 85 | 0.373 | 0.112 |
| 95 | 0.339 | 0.112 |

## 6.1. The Calcaneal Quantitative Ultrasound Studies

One of the earliest studies using quantitative ultrasound to investigate the effect of pregnancy on maternal BMD involved a cross sectional study of 45 first trimester, 56 second trimester, and 129 third trimester women. Speed of sound (SOS) and bone ultrasound attenuation (BUA) values were measured at the os calcis using a generic ultrasound device, and a relational stiffness variable was used as indicator for bone quality. Statistically significant reductions in SOS, BUA and stiffness values were observed during the third trimester as compared to first and second trimester. It was concluded that a linear reduction of ultrasound BMD was observed throughout pregnancy [28]. However, the cross-sectional nature of the data has made detailed interpretation of the magnitude of BMD loss difficult.

In another small Japanese study, 28 pregnant women were followed longitudinally from early pregnancy to up to five years postpartum (maximum). BMD was measured by ultrasonic bone densitometry of the os calcis at early pregnancy, one week postpartum and at six-month intervals thereafter. Stiffness was calculated from the combined values of SOS and BUA. It was found that the BMD in women with 0-1 and 2-6 months lactation duration returned to baseline levels within 1 and 1.5 years postpartum. In women with lactation of 8-12 months, the BMD returned to baseline within 4 years post delivery. The BMD in women with subsequent delivery within 1 year after weaning showed an overall decrease in BMD in the subsequent delivery. The authors concluded that the BMD loss during pregnancy and lactation returned to baseline within 4 years postpartum, depending on the lactation period and the length of time from weaning to the next delivery, but not the actual lactational period [29]. Despite the small sample size in this study, a follow –up of up to 5 years post-delivery was remarkable. There was no data on weight changes during the years of follow-up in the subjects, which could also contribute to the BMD changes. Also the problem of reproducibility and consistency of the BMD measurements repeated in the same individual over long time intervals required further evaluation.

A population based longitudinal study of 307 pregnant British women was performed from early to late pregnancy measuring the left calcaneous using quantitative ultrasound. A significant decline in both SOS and BUA during pregnancy was confirmed. Those who were pregnant for the first time ($p=0.001$), those who had low milk intake pre-pregnancy ($p=0.01$) and those with reduced fat mass ($p=0.01$) showed the greatest decline in calcaneal bone measurements. Women who were pregnant over winter months also had greater losses in the calcaneous ($p=0.02$). It was concluded that maternal life style, fat stores and seasonality of early pregnancy could influence calcaneal BMD loss during pregnancy. The authors believed that the findings supported a role for vitamin D supplementation of women pregnant in winter months, especially in those with low calcium intake who were pregnant for the first time [30].

## 6.2. The Phalangeal Quantitative Ultrasound Studies

A longitudinal study in 40 pregnant women used ultrasonographic bone propagation velocity in the proximal phalanges of fingers 2 to 5 (using the DBM Sonic 1200) together with biochemical markers of bone remodeling in all three trimesters of pregnancy. Ultrasonographic bone propagation was lower in the second and third trimesters of pregnancy ($p < 0.0001$) compared with the respective preceding trimesters. Tartrate resistant acid phosphatase and alkaline phosphatase levels increased significantly ($p < 0.0001$) in parallel with the ultrasound bone propagation decrease. It was concluded that pregnancy was accompanied by a reduction in ultrasound bone propagation velocity that was greater in women with low calcium intake [31]. The coefficient of variation for ultrasound bone propagation velocity was 0.7%. The authors remarked that they have used ultrasound velocity instead of bone velocity attenuation (BUA) because of the lower coefficient of variation with the former technique. However, it could also be seen that despite the lower coefficient of variation for bone velocity measurements, the magnitude of change for SOS parameters was also much smaller compared to BUA measurements, and thus the percentage error of measurement also tend to increase. The problem is apparently intrinsic to using phalangeal ultrasound, as conventionally only SOS measurements are used for this site.

In another study using phalangeal ultrasound, amplitude dependent SOS (AD-SOS) was measured by quantitative ultrasound in 100 healthy white pregnant women and compared with the same number of age-mated, white non-pregnant women. Bone ultrasound velocity was measured at the distal metaphysis of the proximal phalanges of the non-dominant hand from the second to the fifth finger, using the DBM Sonic Bone Profile 1200. In a subgroup of 50 subjects, longitudinal evaluation throughout the pregnancy was performed. A significant reduction of AD-SOS was observed during pregnancy, falling progressively from first to third trimester (first trimester 2118+/- 46 m/s, second trimester 2085 +/- 49m/s, third trimester 2081 +/- 51 m/s). These values in pregnant women were all significantly lower than the values for controls (2170 +/- 55 m/s). There was a negative correlation with body mass index ($r = -0.31$) and a positive correlation with daily calcium intake ($r = 0.33$). Increased levels of urinary markers for bone resorption confirmed an increase in bone turnover [32]. Thus, the results of this study were compatible with the observation of progressive fall in BMD during pregnancy. However, QUS of the phalanges measured more of cortical bone rather than trabecular bone, the magnitude of changes of the former being theoretically much lower in pregnancy as compared to trabecular bone. Thus, it can be seen that the magnitude of fall in AD-SOS demonstrated in this study was only in the range of 1.7 to 2 % from first to third trimester, in contrast to the 3-6% changes using os calcis QUS.

Another similar study also used the DBM Sonic 1200 quantitative ultrasound device to measure the AD–SOS (m/s) of the phalanges longitudinally in the first, second and third trimester in 48 normal pregnant women, and attempted to correlate the findings to fetal and newborn growth. Laboratory investigations were also performed serially, including total serum calcium, total alkaline phosphatase, and phosphate. The hypothesis was that fetal growth and sizes of the newborn could have a direct influence on bone and mineral status in pregnancy. It was found that AD-SOS decreased significantly ($p < 0.0001$) and alkaline phosphatase increased significantly in the second and third trimester of pregnancy ($p < 0.01$). A decrease in AD-SOS greater than the least significant change (LSC) was observed in 22 females (46%) during pregnancy. Changes in alkaline phosphatase correlated significantly with the changes in AD-SOS ($r = -0.31$). However, there were no significant correlations between fetal ultrasonographic measurement parameters (including the femur length and biparietal diameter) and newborn size with changes in AD-SOS. The authors concluded that the study revealed considerable changes in maternal bone and mineral status in normal pregnancy, and confirmed that in a significant proportion of these women, a gradual fall in bone density was evident from first to third trimester [33]. The failure to draw any definite association between the maternal quantitative ultrasound parameters and fetal or newborn growth parameters would be expected, however, both because of the small sample size and the large number of confounding variables that would influence fetal growth apart from maternal bone status.

A very similar German study also performed quantitative ultrasound of the phalanges using a similar device in 60 healthy pregnant women and again demonstrated a significant reduction, from first through second to third trimester, of the amplitude-dependent SOS ($p =< 0.001$) and the bone transmission time ( $p =< 0.001$). The decrease in these values was found to have a large influence on the T scores and Z scores, but was independent of other osteoporosis-related risk factors and the increase in body weight across the trimesters [34].

Finally, another recent study also used quantitative ultrasound of the phalanges using a similar protocol and studied longitudinal changes in AD-SOS and bone transmission time from the first to second to third trimester in 59 pregnant women, of which 38 were nulliparous and 28 were multiparous. Once again, the results confirmed a significant reduction of these parameters in the third trimester, and the T-scores and Z-scores also decreased more rapidly from the second to third trimester. When comparing nulliparous to multiparous women, it was found that the AD-SOS was lower at the beginning of pregnancy in the multiparous group, then increased from first to second trimester, and then decreased again from second to third trimester, similar to nulliparous women.

On the other hand, bone transmission time showed little variation in multiparous women between first and second trimester, and at term, the values were higher than the group of nulliparous women. The authors concluded that that there was an important reduction in these QUS variables probably coinciding with an increase of remodeling with bone demineralization in the third trimester of pregnancy. They also commented that there could be a difference in the bone metabolism changes between nulliparous and multiparous women [35].

# 7. Longitudinal Cohort Studies Using Quantitative USG of the os calcis on BMD Changes in Pregnancy

In the past years, we have performed a series of observational studies using QUS of the os calcis to study BMD changes in pregnancy in detail. The QUS BMD measurements were performed at the os calcis bilaterally at booking between 10 to 18 weeks, and then in late third trimester at 36-38 weeks. All measurements were done using the Sahara Clinical Bone Sonometer system (Hologic) [Figure 1], a waterless portable system that involved direct contact of the probe with the heel through elastomer pads and a coupling gel. The system was able to generate a simulated bone mineral density (BMD) value apart from other proprietary values, and this was used in the subsequent analysis for calculations. The coefficient of variation for the estimated heel BMD value was 2-3% as quoted by the manufacturer. The mean values of the left and right os calcis BMD was used in subsequent calculations. In addition to weight, body fat percentage assay was also performed in each of these occasions using a Tanita 500 bio-impedance system. The serial BMD findings were then correlated with the clinical data of each patient after her delivery, including significant antenatal and perinatal complications, as well as the immediate pregnancy outcome.

In a cohort of 780 women, the difference in BMD across serial measurements during pregnancy was highly significant, and a mean fall of BMD of 0.40 g/cm was demonstrable from early pregnancy to late first trimester, which represented around 6% of the early pregnancy BMD values. A regression model of quantitative variables showed that fat accumulation ($p = 0.03$) and early pregnancy BMD values ($p < 0.001$) were significant factors associated with BMD loss in pregnancy. This large cohort was thus able to show that quantitative ultrasound was a viable tool for monitoring the changes in BMD in pregnancy [36].

Using the same protocol, the BMD changes in gestational diabetic and non-diabetic pregnancies were evaluated in a cohort of 480 patients, of which 96 had gestational diabetes

(GDM) diagnosed according to the WHO criteria. The mean BMD loss was higher in diabetic patients as compared to the controls (0.038 Vs 0.025 mg/cm$^2$, p =0.048). However, a regression model of all pregnancies showed that higher fat accumulation was related to lower BMD loss, but diabetic status was not in the equation. While gestational diabetic women had higher BMD loss as compared to non-diabetic women, this was apparently secondary to other anthropometric factors related to dietary treatment of their GMD status rather than directly to the gestational diabetic state [37]. A similar study aiming at comparing the maternal BMD changes in gestational hypertensive and normotensive pregnancies using quantitative ultrasound was also performed in the same cohort. The changes in BMD from early to late pregnancy were compared between those with/ without gestational hypertension. The overall incidence of gestational hypertension was 4.8% of which 1.7% fulfilled the definitions of severe pre-eclampsia. The hypertensive group has marginally higher mean BMD loss as compared to the normotensive group (0.052 g/cm$^2$ Vs 0.037 g/cm$^2$; p =0.037). However, regression analysis models showed that early pregnancy BMD values, early pregnancy fat percentage and fat accumulation in pregnancy were more significant factors affecting BMD loss during pregnancy, while gestational hypertension was not in the equations. The development of gestational hypertensive disorders apparently does not have any significant impact on bone mineral density changes during pregnancy [38]. Thus, both the studies on gestational diabetes and hypertension showed that anthropometric characteristics of the pregnant women were more important factors that influenced the BMD loss in pregnancy, rather than the antenatal complications themselves.

We then proceeded on to evaluate whether back pain symptoms in pregnancy are associated with BMD changes. Patients in this cohort were surveyed for back pain symptoms they experienced during pregnancy in the early postpartum period. The self-reported back pain symptoms were then correlated with BMD changes. Of a total of 463 patients, 231 (49.8 %) reported one or more episodes of significant back pain during pregnancy. Those with back pain symptoms have higher mean BMD loss at the os calcis during pregnancy compared to those without back pain (0.038 g/cm2 Vs 0.029 g/cm2; p=0.012). A logistic regression model showed that weight gain in pregnancy and BMD loss in pregnancy were significantly associated with the development of back pain symptoms. Thus, those with back pain symptoms in pregnancy apparently had a greater fall in BMD values at the os calcis, supporting the hypothesis that BMD changes could have an aetiological role in back pain during pregnancy [39].

We then evaluated whether bone mineral density (BMD) changes in women engaged in active exercises during pregnancy would be different from non-exercising women. A total of 24 physically active women with singleton pregnancies undergoing active physical training of over 10 hours per week at 20 weeks gestation and beyond (mean 13.1 hrs, SD 3.3) were compared to 94 non-exercising low risk women. A marginal fall in BMD of 0.015 g/cm$^2$ (SD 0.034) was demonstrable from early to late gestation in the exercising women, which was significantly lower than that of non-exercising women (0.041 g/cm$^2$; SD 0.042; p = 0.005).

Logistic regression models confirmed that active exercises in pregnancy were significantly associated with absence of or less BMD loss in pregnancy. In women actively engaged in physical training during pregnancy, the physiological fall in BMD during pregnancy was apparently less compare to those that were not regularly exercising [40].

A postpartum study was then performed to evaluate the use of QUS of the os calcis to monitor BMD changes after delivery. The initial cohort of low risk patients that were studied for BMD changes during pregnancy were invited for follow-up and review around 2 years after their delivery, and QUS measurements were repeated 24-28 months after their delivery. A total of 95 patients completed the study, of which 55(57.8%) were primiparous and 40 (42%) were multiparous. A mean fall in BMD of 0.0389 g/cm$^2$ was demonstrable from early to late gestation. The mean BMD difference between the 2-year assessment and early pregnancy (Δ BMD) was -0.008g/cm$^2$. Δ BMD was negligible for multiparous women compared to a small loss in primiparous women (0.0006 Vs -0014 g/cm$^2$, p=0.026). There were no significant differences in Δ BMD between those that lactated for over 16 weeks (n=35) and those that did not (n=60). A logistic regression model showed the extent of BMD loss during pregnancy and pregnancy weight gain were significant factors associated with BMD changes 24 months after delivery. We concluded that BMD loss during pregnancy that was detectable by quantitative ultrasound at the os calcis has largely recovered at 24 months after delivery [41].

Using the cohort with back pain symptoms in pregnancy, we then evaluated whether persistence of back pain symptoms 2 years after pregnancy could be associated with BMD changes as measured by quantitative USG of the os calcis. Thus, the cohort recruited for the initial back pain study was followed up and surveyed for persistent back pain symptoms 24 to 28 months after the index pregnancy. Os calcis BMD was measured by quantitative ultrasound and compared with the BMD values during pregnancy. A cohort of 60 women who had reported significant back pain symptoms in their index pregnancy completed a 24-28 months follow-up survey and BMD reassessment. Persistence of significant back pain symptoms was seen in 24 (40%) of this cohort.

These women had higher BMD loss during pregnancy compared to those without further pain (0.047 Vs 0.030 g/cm$^2$; p =0.03). Those that remained pain free after pregnancy appeared to have completely recovered their BMD loss in pregnancy, while those with persistent pain had marginally lower BMD values (ΔBMD 0.0078 Vs 0.025 g/cm$^2$; p =0.023) compared to their early pregnancy values. Thus, we concluded that persistence of back pain symptoms after pregnancy could be related to an inability to recover fully from BMD loss during the index pregnancy [42].

## 8. BMD Changes in Pregnancy and Its Association to Bone Health in Later Life

All women lose bone after menopause. The main determinants of postmenopausal bone loss giving rise to osteoporosis would be the rate of bone loss and the peak bone mass [14]. The presence of osteoporosis and its severity will determine the risks osteoporotic fractures in later life [Table 3]. Pregnancy and lactation are common physiological events that could affect peak bone mass and thus the development of osteoporosis later in life. However, most previous epidemiological studies have failed to show consistent results of an association between pregnancy, parity and BMD. These studies can broadly be divided into those examining short term effects of pregnancy on BMD within a few years after pregnancy and lactation, and longer term effects in terms of bone health in menopausal life.

**Table 3. Diagnostic criteria for osteoporosis according to BMD T-scores WHO 2003 criteria**

| Category | Definition of bone density |
|---|---|
| Normal | BMD or BMC values no more than 1 SD below the young adult mean value |
| Low bone mass or osteopenia | BMD or BMC values between 1 and 2.5 SD below the young adult mean value |
| Osteoporosis | BMD or BMC values more than 2.5 SD below the young adult mean value |
| Severe osteoporosis ( or established osteoporosis) | BMD or BMC values more than 2.5 SD below the young adult mean value in the presence of one or more fragility fractures |

## 8.1. Short Term Effects of Pregnancy and Lactation on Bone Health

A study using DXA of hip BMD on 60 normal women before conception and then during the subsequent pregnancy and up to one year after delivery showed that there was a fall in BMD at the spine (1.53%), total hip (1.15%) and trochanter (3.90%) but not the femoral neck. After delivery, the women who breast-fed showed a significant fall in BMD at all sites, while those who bottle-fed had increased or maintained BMD at all sites. It was concluded that lactation posed a risk factor for BMD loss, with 47% of lactating women losing over 5% of BMD at either the lumbar spine and trochanter. However, at one year after delivery, most women had returned to within 5% of pre-conceptional values [43].

In a cross-sectional study of 119 adolescents ranging from 12-20 years of age, in which 30 had history of a full term pregnancy, areal and volumetric BMD studies showed that the proportion with abnormal Z-scores were the same between those with or without pregnancy history and there was no association between pregnancy history and low bone mass [44]. The authors suggested that adolescent pregnancy has no impact on acquisition of peak bone mass and should not represent a risk factor for osteoporosis in future.

To study the effects of lactation on BMD, a cohort of 308 women who lactated for 6 months followed by 1-month weaning period were compared to a control group of non-lactating women during the first 18 months postpartum. Progressive decrease in BMD as measured radiologically at the spine and radius was seen in the lactating women over the first 6 months, followed by recovery up to levels that at 18 months were higher than the baseline. In non-lactating women, BMD also increased progressively after delivery, and at 18 months postpartum, had increased by 1.1 to 1.9% compared to baseline. The authors concluded that lactating women with longer amenorrhoea initially lost more bone, but also gained significantly after resumption of menses, so that at 18 months there were little differences between the two groups [45].

In another study, the influence of pregnancy on BMD was evaluated using DXA in a group of healthy women postpartum with age matched controls and compared with healthy women with a maximum of two pregnancies to test the effects of multiparity on BMD. It was found that those with multiple previous pregnancies did not have lower BMD, and those with prolonged lactation showed initial BMD loss but recovered within 5 months of weaning. It was concluded that neither an extended lactational period nor repeated previous pregnancies could be used as risk factors for predicting future osteoporosis [46].

Thus, it can be seen that in most of these studies, while BMD loss can be observed with pregnancy and lactation, the loss normally would recover within a short period of time after weaning. Pregnancy is not shown to be, and should not be regarded as a risk factor for subsequent osteoporosis.

## 8.2. Parity and Long Term Menopausal Bone Health –The Positive Effects

Many studies have reported a positive association of parity with BMD in menopausal age. In a large cohort of 2230 white women aged 65 or above, radial BMD as measured by single photon absorptiometry was correlated with parity, lactation and menstruation history. It was found that the number of births, duration of menstrual bleeding, age of menarche, and years menstruating were significant independent predictors of postmenopausal BMD. A 1.4% increase in distal radius BMD was observed with each additional birth, but no difference in BMD was demonstrated for women who breast-fed and women who did not [47]. In another cohort of 580 postmenopausal women, similar correlations between reproductive factors and BMD of the spine, hip and radius were made. It was found that the number of pregnancies were more strongly associated with increased BMD on femoral neck and total radius, but not the spine, trochanter or total body. Breast feeding duration, duration of oral contraceptive use and premenopausal amenorrhoea were found to have no association with BMD [48].

When a cohort of 83 female twin pairs who were discordant for ever having been pregnant were screened for their BMD by formal DXA, no significant within-pair differences in unadjusted BMD or BMD adjusted for age, height, and fat mass at the lumbar spine or total hip or in total body bone mineral content was seen [49]. When 498 twins were studied with regard to parity number, there was no significant within-pair difference in measures of bone mineral or body composition related to the within-pair differences in the number of pregnancies, which ranged from 1 to 3. The authors concluded there were no long term detrimental effects of pregnancy or breast feeding on bone mineral measures [49].

In addition, a cross –sectional study of 168 Hutterite women aged 40-80 with parity ranging from zero to 16, it was found that high parity was associated with increased radial torsional bending strength and femoral neck size. The authors suggested that the greater femoral neck size, without higher BMD, might explain the reduced hip fracture risks among these women with high parity [50]. Thus, the positive effects of parity on bone may be mediated not through BMD but bone size.

## 8.3. Parity and Long Term Menopausal Bone Health – The Negative Effects

However, neutral or negative associations with parity were also repeatedly reported. In a special cohort of 426 Old Order Amish women with particularly high parity aged 40 or older, it was found that the high parity is associated with increased hip BMD, largely mediated by a high body mass index in these women. The benefit of high parity on BMD appeared to be lost soon after the menopausal transition, so that parity apparently posed neither a detrimental nor beneficial effect on long term bone health [51]. Similarly, in a cohort of 509 postmenopausal women, correlation of reproductive factors and BMD at four sites showed the BMD values of the spine and femur decreases with an increasing number of pregnancies, particularly at the 40-59 year old age group as compared to the older 60-80 age group. The authors concluded from their data that parity of five or above was indicative of a risk factor for postmenopausal fractures [52].

Another study of 303 postmenopausal Turkish women correlated their BMD values with age at menarche, age at first pregnancy, number of pregnancies and total breast feeding time. A negative correlation was seen between the number of parities and BMD. The BMD values decreased as the number of pregnancies increased, particularly in those with more than five parities, as well as with increasing age at first pregnancy. Also, women who had 5 or more abortions were also found to have significantly lower spine BMD values compared to women who had no abortions or fewer abortions. Thus, it was concluded that increased risk of osteoporosis was associated with increased number of pregnancies and higher age at first pregnancy [53].

In a study to screen 2080 postmenopausal women using quantitative ultrasound of the calcaneus, nulliparous women were compared to parous women grouped according to the number of births, and those who had never breast fed were compared to women who had. No statistically significant associations were found between the quantitative ultrasound variables and parity or breast feeding, even after controlling for confounding variables in matched pair or regression analysis [54].

## 8.4. Fracture Risks and Parity

Hypothetically, there could be an increased risk of sustaining fractures during pregnancy or in the postpartum period when BMD is still low and before the woman regain her former level of BMD. However, except in the case of pathological osteoporosis associated with pregnancy, most women still have a BMD of sufficiently high level to withstand fractures [25], and to date there have been no formal studies on the incidence of fractures or fracture risks during the months of pregnancy.

On the other hand, the notion that fracture incidences in mid life for women with multiple parities was no different from that of nulliparous women has been supported by several older studies, including a longitudinal study of 9704 American women over 65 years of age [55], a cross-sectional study of 2086 women with a hip fracture from fourteen European centres and another 3532 controls [56], and the European Vertebral Osteoporosis Study (EVOS), a longitudinal study including 6646 women aged 50-79 years [57]. All of these large epidemiological studies have not shown any significant differences in the incidence of fractures in non-parous versus parous women.

More directly, the relationship between parity, lactation and the occurrence of hip fractures were investigated in several epidemiological studies. In a case controlled study of 174 white women with a confirmed first hip fracture and selected age matched controls, it was found that ever having a live birth was associated with reduced odds of hip fracture. When body mass index was also controlled, each birth was associated on average with 9% reduction in the odds of hip fracture (OR =0.92) [58].

As part of the Leisure World study [59], 8,600 postmenopausal women were evaluated for risk factors for hip fractures. Together with other factors such as active exercises and high body mass index, higher parity, late age of menarche, long menstrual cycle length and oestrogen therapy (particularly recent users) were associated with reduction in hip fracture risk while cigarette smoking increased the risk. Similarly, in the Dubbo Osteoporosis Epidemiological Study, data from 1091 women in their seventies also showed that high parity and longer duration of exposure to oestrogen, either through natural menstruation or postmenopausal hormonal replacement, have protective effects on BMD and were associated with a reduced incidence of atraumatic fracture [60].

A Swedish survey amongst postmenopausal women aged 50-81 years also showed that the risk of hip fractures were reduced by 10 % per child, and 5% per child even after multivariate adjustment. After parity was considered, there was no association of duration of lactation period with fracture risk. The authors concluded that parity is a modestly associated with a reduced hip fracture risk among women who had not used oral contraceptives previously [61]. A cross-sectional survey of 2045 elderly Danish twins aged 75-98 was performed to study the association between different aspects of their reproductive history and hip fractures. It was found that having no children was associated with a higher risk of hip fracture compared to having at least one child, and with similar results in a prospective survey of 3057 twins aged 66-99 years followed for a total of 29,112 years [62]. Finally, a study of 1855 postmenopausal Hispanic women in Colombia, many being of high parity, also showed higher BMD and lower risks of fractures (OR 0.41) among multiparous women compared to nulliparous ones [63].

In contrast to using BMD as the end-parameter, when both positive and negative effects of pregnancy on menopausal bone density has been reported, it can be seen that the literature appears to be consistent that when analyzing fracture incidences and risks. Overall, pregnancy appears to be a protective or neutral factor against menopausal fractures.

# Conclusion

The data presented in this chapter consistently supported the finding of a substantial fall in BMD at various bone sites during pregnancy, and it is also apparent that for most women, such BMD loss would recover within a few years after their delivery. The long term impact of pregnancy, parity and lactation on subsequent menopausal osteoporosis has been debated for a long time, but the general consensus that the transient BMD loss observed in pregnancy should not be detrimental to bone health in the long run seems to be well accepted. Thus, in the majority of women, monitoring of BMD changes in pregnancy, be it by quantitative ultrasound or other radiological methods, would be unnecessary and should not be clinically useful. However, there are certain “high risk” women that such BMD monitoring should be considered, which would also be clinically relevant for management. These include women with significant back pain in pregnancy, women with specific medical disorders in pregnancy that would predispose to subsequent osteoporosis and those at risk of transient osteoporosis of pregnancy. Future directions in studying changes in BMD in pregnancy should be focused on these high risk groups.

## Summary Points

1) The maternal skeleton remains the most important source of calcium to the fetus during pregnancy, with a full term neonate containing around 30 g calcium.
2) Normal adaptative responses during pregnancy and lactation allow for adequate delivery of minerals to the fetus or infant, while at the same time protecting to a certain degree the maternal skeleton.
3) Earlier studies have utilized radiological methods such as single-photon absorptiometry (SPA) and dual energy X-ray absorptiometry (DXA), which are usually regarded as inadvisable during pregnancy because of risks of radiation exposure.
4) Quantitative ultrasonography (QUS) offers an inexpensive, non-invasive, radiation-free method by which to assess BMD and bone quality during pregnancy.
5) The use of QUS for monitoring BMD changes in pregnancy and after delivery has often been challenged because of the lower precision of such techniques with a larger coefficient of variation as compared to radiological methods. However, the current data have confirmed that the changes in BMD during pregnancy were consistently greater than the least minimal change measurable by such systems, supporting the validity for using QUS for monitoring.
6) The current data on QUS to survey BMD changes in pregnancy basically used either calcaneal/os calcis or phalangeal measurements. Os calcis measurements are preferable as this site contains mainly trabecular bone and BMD changes are more significantly observable.
7) Both radiological and ultrasound methods have shown a consistent pattern of loss of BMD from either preconception or early pregnancy to late pregnancy and early postpartum period of around 3-6%, depending on the bone sites measured and the methods used.
8) Form QUS studies, it was found that the degree of BMD loss in pregnancy could be related to body weight, body fat composition, pre-pregnancy / early pregnancy BMD values, other antenatal complications and exercising levels. Higher BMD loss during pregnancy may be related to higher rates of back pain, and the incomplete recovery of this BMD loss after delivery could be related to persistent back pain symptoms.
9) While BMD loss can be observed with pregnancy and lactation, the loss normally would recover within a short period of time. Pregnancy is not shown to be, and should not be regarded as a risk factor for subsequent osteoporosis.
10) Epidemiological data have shown that parity and lactation do not have significant detrimental effects on bone health in later life. Pregnancy appears to be a protective or neutral factor against menopausal fractures.

## References

[1] Purdie DW, Aaron JE, Selby PL. Bone histology and mineral homeostasis in human pregnancy. *Br. J. Obstet. Gynaecol.* 1988; 95: 849-854.

[2] Sowers M. Pregnancy and lactation as risk factors for subsequent bone loss and osteoporosis. *J. Bone Miner Res.* 1996: 11: 1052-1060.

[3] Ulrich U, Miller PB, Eyre DR, Chestnut CH, Schlebusch H, Soules MR. Bone remodeling and bone mineral density during pregnancy. *Arch. Gynecol. Obstet.* 2003; 268: 309-316.

[4] Hosking DJ. Calcium homeostasis in pregnancy. *Clin. Endocrinol.* 1996; 45: 1-6.

[5] Gertner J, Coustan D, Kliger A, Mallette L, Ravin N, Broadus A. Pregnancy as a state of physiologic absorptive hypercalciuria. *Am. J. Med.* 1986; 81: 451-456.

[6] Kent G, Price R, Gutteridge D, Rossman K, Smith M, Allen J, Hickling C, Blakeman S. The efficiency of intestinal calcium absorption is increased in late pregnancy but not established lactation. *Calcif. Tissue Int.* 1991; 48: 293-295.

[7] Kent G, Price R, Gutteridge D, Allen J, Rosman K, Smith M, Bhagat C, Wilson S, Retallack R. Effect of pregnancy and lactation on maternal bone mass and calcium metabolism. *Osteoporosis* 1993 (Suppl 1), S44-S47.

[8] Shahtaheri SM, Aaron JE, Johnson DR, Purdie DW. Changes in trabecular bone architecture in women during pregnancy. *Br. J. Obstet. Gynaecol.* 1999; 106: 432-438.

[9] Christiansen C, Rodbro P, Heinild B. Unchanged total body calcium in normal human pregnancy. *Acta Obstet. Gynecol. Scand.* 1976; 55: 141-143.

[10] Sowers M, Crutchfield M, Jannausch M, Updike S, Corton G. A prospective evaluation of bone mineral change in pregnancy. *Obstet. Gynecol.* 1991; 77: 841-845.

[11] Matsumoto I, Kosha S, Noguchi S, Kojima N, Oki T, Douchi T, Nagata Y. Changes in bone mineral density in pregnancy and postpartum women. *J. Obstet. Gynaecol.* (Tokyo) 1995; 21: 419-425.

[12] Drinkwater B, Chestnut C. Bone density changes during pregnancy and lactation in active women: a longitudinal study. *Bone Miner* 1991; 14: 153-160.

[13] More C, Bettembuk P, Bhattoa H, Balogh A. The effects of pregnancy and lactation on bone mineral density. *Osteoporosis Int.* 2001; 12: 732-737.

[14] Kaur M, Pearson D, Godber I, Lawson N, Baker P, Hosking D. Longitudinal changes in bone mineral density during normal pregnancy. *Bone* 2003; 32: 449-454.

[15] Phillips AJ, Ostere SJ, Smith R. Pregnancy-associated osteoporosis: does the skeleton recover? *Osteoporosis Int.* 2000; 11: 449-454.

[16] Naylor KE, Iqbal P, Fledelius C, Fraser RB, Eastell R. The effect of pregnancy on bone density and bone turnover. *J. Bone Mineral Res.* 2000; 15: 129-137.

[17] Lamke B, Brundin J, Moberg P. Changes of bone mineral content during pregnancy and lactation. *Acta Obstet. Gynecol. Scand.* 1977; 56: 217-219.

[18] Wisser J, Florio I, Neff M, Konig V, Huch R, Huch A, von Mandach U. Changes in bone density and metabolism in pregnancy. *Acta Obstet. Gynecol. Scand.* 2005; 84: 349-354.

[19] Liu A, Qiu L, Chen YM, Su YX. Effect of milk and calcium supplementation on bone density and bone turnover in pregnant Chinese women: a randomized controlled trial. *Arch. Gynecol. Obstet.* 2011; 283: 205-211.

[20] Olausson H, Laskey MA, Goldberg GR, Prentice A. Changes on bone mineral status and bone size during pregnancy and the influence of body weight and calcium intake. *Am. J. Clin. Nutr.* 2008; 88: 1032-1039.

[21] Karlsson MK, Ahlborg HK, Karlsson C. Maternity and bone mineral density. *Acta Orthopaedica* 2005; 76: 2-13.

[22] Uematsu N, Nakayama Y, Shirai Y, Tamai K, Hashiguchi H, Banzai Y. Transient osteoporosis of the hip during pregnancy. *J. Nippon Med. Sch.* 2000; 67: 459-463.

[23] Lloyd JM, Lewis M, Jones A. Transient osteoporosis of the knee in pregnancy. *J. Knee Surg.* 2006; 19: 121-123.

[24] Willis-Owen CA, Daurka JA, Chen A, Lewis A. Bilateral femoral neck fractures due to transient osteoporosis of pregnancy: a case report. *Cases Journal* 2008; 1: 120.

[25] Aynaci O, Kerimoglu S, Ozturk C, Saracoglu M. Bilateral non-traumatic acetabular and femoral neck fractures due to pregnancy-associated osteoporosis. *Arth. Orthop. trauma Surg.* 2008; 128: 313-316.

[26] Spinarelli A, Patella V, Speciale D, Petrera M, Vittore D, Pesce V, Patella S. Hip fracture in a patient affected by transient osteoporosis of the femoral head during the last trimester of pregnancy. *Orthopedics* 2009; 32: 365.

[27] Nassiri DK. Ultrasound bone densitometry – real or imaginary? *Ultrasound Obstet Gynecol.* 1999; 14: 87-91.

[28] Paparella P, Giorgino R, Maglione A, Lorusso D, Scripa P, Del-Bosco A, Mancuso S. Maternal ultrasound bone density in normal pregnancy. *Clin. Exp. Obstet. Gynecol.* 1995; 22: 268-278.

[29] Yoneyama K, Ikeda J. Change in maternal bone mineral density during pregnancy and relationship between the density and foetus growth – a prospective study. *Jap J. Public Health* 2000; 47: 661-669.

[30] Javaid MK, Crozier SR, Harvey NC, Taylor P, Inskip HM, Godfrey KM, Cooper C and the Southampton Women's Survey Study Group. Maternal and seasonal predictors of change in calcaneal quantitative ultrasound during pregnancy. *J. Clin. Endocrinol. Metab.* 2005; 90: 5182-5187.

[31] Aguado F, Revilla M, Hernandez ER, Menendez M, Cortes-Prieto J, Villa LF, Rico H. Ultrasonographic bone velocity in pregnancy: a longitudinal study. *Am. J. Obstet. Gynecol.* 1998; 178: 1016-1021.

[32] Tranquilli AL, Giannubilo SR, Corradetti A. Ultrasound measurement of pregnancy induced changes in maternal bone mass: a longitudinal cross-sectional and biochemical study. *Gynecol. Endocrinol.* 2004; 18: 258-262.

[33] Pluskiewicz W, Drozdzowska B, Stolecki M. Quantitative ultrasound at the hand phalanges in pregnancy: a longitudinal study. *Ultrasound Med. Biol.* 2004; 30: 1373-1378.

[34] Hellmeyer L, Ossendorf A, Ziller V, Tekesin I, Schmidt S, Hadji P. Quantitative ultrasonometry of the phalanges during pregnancy: a longitudinal study. *Climateric* 2006B; 9: 446-451.

[35] Martina MD, Biasioli A, Vascotto L, Rinuncini D, Menegato AA, Liva S, Londero AP, Driul L, Marchesoni D. Bone ultrasonometry measurement in pregnancy. *Arch. Gynecol. Obstet.* 2010; 281: 401-407.

[36] To WWK, Wong MWN, Leung TW: Relationship between bone mineral density changes in pregnancy and maternal and pregnancy characteristics: a longitudinal study. *Acta Obstet. Gynecol. Scand.* 2003; 82: 820-827.

[37] To WWK, Wong MWN (2008). Bone mineral density changes in gestational diabetic pregnancies: a longitudinal study using quantitative ultrasound measurements of the os calcis. *Gynecological Endocrinology;* 24: 519-525.

[38] To WWK, Wong MWN (2010). Bone mineral density changes in pregnancies with gestational hypertension: a longitudinal study using quantitative ultrasound measurements. *Arch. Gynecol. Obstet.* 2011; 284: 39-44. *Erratum* 2011; 284:45.

[39] To WWK, Wong MWN. Back pain symptoms and bone mineral density changes in pregnancy as measured by quantitative ultrasound. *Gynecol. Obstet Invest.* 2009; 67: 36-41.

[40] To WWK, Wong MWN. Bone Mineral Density changes during pregnancy in actively exercising women as measured by quantitative ultrasound. *Arch. Obstet. Gynecol.* 2012; 286: 357-363.

[41] To WWK, Wong MWN. Changes in bone mineral density of the os calcis as measured by quantitative ultrasound during pregnancy and 24 months after delivery. *Aust. NZ J. Obstet. Gynecol.* 2011; 51: 166-171.

[42] To WWK, Wong MWN. Persistence of back pain symptoms after pregnancy and bone mineral density changes as measured by quantitative ultrasound – a two year longitudinal follow up study. *BioMed. Central Musculoskeletal* 2011: 12: 55.

[43] Pearson D, Kaur M, San P, Lawson N, Baker P, Hosking D. Recovery of pregnancy mediated bone loss during lactation. *Bone* 2004; 570-578.

[44] Miglioli L, Costa-paiva L, De Lourenco LS, Morais SS, Lopes De Lima MC, Pinto-Neto AM. The association of pregnancy history with areal and volumetric bone mineral density in adolescence. *Osteoporos Int.* 2007; 18: 101-108.

[45] Polatti F, Capuzzo E, Viazzo F, Colleoni R, Klersy C. Bone mineral changes during and after lactation. *Obstet. Gynecol.* 1999; 94: 52-56.

[46] Karlsson C, Obrant K, Karlsson M. Pregnancy and lactation confer reversible bone loss in humans. *Osteoporosis Int.* 2001; 12: 823-834.

[47] Fox KM, Magaziner J, Sherwin R, Scott JC, Plato CC, Nevitt M, Cummings S. Reproductive correlates of bone mass in elderly women. Study of Osteoporotic Fractures Research Group. *J. Bone Miner Res.* 1993; 8: 901-908.

[48] Grainge MJ, Coupland CAC, cliffe SJ, Chilvers CED, Hosking DJ. Reproductive, menstrual and menopausal factors: which are associated with bone mineral density in early postmenopausal women? *Osteoporosis Int.* 2001; 12: 777-787.

[49] Paton LM, Alexander JL, Nowson CA, Margerison C, Frame MG, Kaymakei B, Wark JD. Pregnancy and lactation have no long-term deleterious effect on measures of bone mineral in healthy women: a twin study. *Am. J. Clin. Nutr.* 2003; 77:707-714.

[50] Specker B, Binkley T. High parity is associated with increased bone size and strength. *Osteoporos Int.* 2005; 16: 1969-1974.

[51] Streeten EA, Ryan KA, McBride DJ, Pollin TI, Shuldiner AR. The relationship between parity and bone mineral density in women characterized by a homogeneous lifestyle and high parity. *J. Clin. Endocrinol. Metab.* 2005; 90: 4536-4541.

[52] Gur A, Nas K, Cevik R, Sarac AJ, Ataoglu S, Karakoc M. Influence of number of pregnancies on bone mineral density in postmenopausal women of different age groups. *J. Bone Miner Metab.* 2003; 21: 234-241.

[53] Ozdemir F, Demirbag D, Rodoplu M. Reproductive factors affecting the bone mineral density in postmenopausal women. *Tohoku J. Exp. Med.* 2005; 205: 277-285.

[54] Hadji P, Ziller V, Kalder M, Gottschalk M, Hellmeyer L, Hars O, Schmidt S, Schulz KD. Influence of pregnancy and breast-feeding on quantitative ultrasonometry of bone in postmenopausal women. *Climateric* 2002; 5: 277-285.

[55] Cummings SR, Nevitt MC, Browner WS, Stone K, Fox KM, Ensnid KE, Cauley J, Black D, Vogt M. Risk factors for hip fracture in white women. Study of Osteoporotic Fractures Research Group. *New Engl. J. Med.* 1995; 332: 767-763.

[56] O'Neill TW, Silman AJ, Naves Diaz M, Cooper C, Kanis J, Felsenberg D. Influence of hormonal and reproductive factors on risk of vertebral deformity in European women. Eurpoean Vertebral Osteoporosis Study Group. *Osteoporosis Int.* 1997; 7: 72-78.

[57] Paganini-Hill A, Chao A, Ross RK, Henderson BE. Exercise and other factors in the prevention of hip fracture: the Leisure World Study. *Epidemiology* 1991; 2: 16-25.

[58] Hoffman S, Grisso JA, Kelsey JL, Gammon MD, O'Brien LA. Parity, lactation and hip fracture. *Osteoporos Int.* 1993; 3: 171-176.

[59] Johnell O, Gullberg B, Kanis JA, Allander E, elffors I, Dequeker J, Dilsen G, Gennari C, Lopes Vaz A, Lyritis G. Risk factors for hip fracture in European women : the MEDOS study. Mediterranean Osteoporosis Study. *J. Bone Miner Res.* 1995; 10: 1802 -1815.

[60] Nguyen TV, Jones G, Sambrook PN, White CP, Kelly PJ, Eisman JA. Effects of estrogen exposure and reproductive factors on bone mineral density and osteoporotic fractures. *J. Clin. Endocrinol. Metab.* 1995; 80: 2709-2714.

[61] Michaelsson K, Baron JA, Farahmand BY, Ljunghall S. Influence of parity and lactation on hip fracture risk. *Am. J. Epidemiol.* 2001; 153: 1166-1172.

[62] Petersen HC, Jeune B, Vaupel JW, Christensen K. Reproduction life history and hip fractures. *Ann. Epidermiol. 2002*; 12: 257-263.

[63] Cure-Cure C, Cure-Ramirez P, Teran E, Lopez-Jaramillo P. Bone mass peak in multiparity and reduced risk of bone-fractures in menopause. *Int. J. Gynaecol. Obstet.* 2002; 76: 285-291.

[64] Jergas M, Schmid G. The role of quantitative ultrasound versus other techniques in osteoporosis assessment. In: Quantitative ultrasound assessment of osteoporosis and bone status. Ed: Njeh CF, Hans D, Fuerst T, Gluer CC, Genant HK. Pub: Martin Dunitz, London 1999. P245-281.

In: Bone Disorders, Screening and Treatment
Editor: Aubrey M. Stone

ISBN: 978-1-63482-155-1


*Chapter 3*

# Development of Vitamin D Deficiency in Obese Individuals Undergoing Bariatric Surgery

*William Hsueh, MD,*[1] *Bikram S. Bal, MD,*[3]
*Timothy R. Shope, MD,*[2] *and Timothy R. Koch, MD*[*1]
[1]Section of Gastroenterology & Hepatology
[2]Center for Advanced Laparoscopic & Bariatric Surgery and Department of Surgery,
MedStar-Washington Hospital Center and Georgetown University School of Medicine,
Washington, DC
[3]Center for Gastrointestinal and Liver Diseases,
Centra Southside, Farmville, VA

## Abstract

Obesity and its related comorbidities have long been shown to have detrimental effects on health. Since dietary and lifestyle interventions are often ineffective in producing sustained weight loss, bariatric surgery has become a major therapeutic option for individuals with medically-complicated obesity.

Micronutrient disorders including vitamin D deficiency are commonly found in individuals before bariatric surgery, perhaps due to inadequate oral intake of vitamin D or due to vitamin D malabsorption. Vitamin D deficiency has been shown to persist after bariatric surgery. Vitamin D deficiency is a major clinical concern since bariatric patients remain at risk for bone diseases, including osteoporosis and osteomalacia.

Increased pre-operative body mass index has been shown in studies to be a risk factor for vitamin D deficiency. Data regarding different bariatric surgical procedures as risk factors for vitamin D deficiency have been conflicting. It has been suggested that

* Correspondence to: Timothy R. Koch, M.D., Professor of Medicine (Gastroenterology), Center for Advanced Laparoscopic & Bariatric Surgery, POB North, Suite 3400, MedStar-Washington Hospital Center and Georgetown University School of Medicine, 106 Irving Street, NW, Washington, DC 20010 United States. Email: timothy.r.koch@medstar.net. Telephone and fax: Telephone: +1-202 8777788; FAX: +1-877 6808198.

patients who have undergone vertical sleeve gastrectomy or adjustable gastric banding have significantly higher vitamin D levels and improvement in vitamin D deficiency when compared to individuals who have undergone Roux-en-Y gastric bypass. Available results suggest that bariatric procedures which emphasize restrictive strategies may initially improve vitamin D deficiency compared to bariatric procedures which utilize restriction and malabsorption.

It has been suggested that the bypass of upper small intestine may promote vitamin D malabsorption. Our studies have however expanded upon prior reports of increased serum levels of folate in individuals with small intestinal bacterial overgrowth. Our results suggest that small intestinal bacterial overgrowth is a potential mechanism to explain post-operative vitamin D deficiency.

Improved understanding of the mechanisms involved in pre-operative vitamin D deficiency and the disorders that inhibit correction of vitamin D deficiency after bariatric surgery should improve the treatment of vitamin D deficiency in individuals who undergo bariatric surgery. Further studies should demonstrate a reduction in the risks of developing osteoporosis and osteomalacia in those individuals who have improved repletion of this important micronutrient.

## Growing International Prevalence of Obesity

The conditions described by overweight and obesity can be defined by an individual's body mass index with overweight represented by a body mass index of 25 to 30 kg/m$^2$, while obesity is defined as a body mass index of >30 kg/m$^2$. The prevalence of overweight and obese people has continued to increase worldwide over the past 3 decades. A recent study in the British literature has summarized worldwide trends in this field of research [1]. It has been estimated that in 2010, the conditions of obesity and overweight were responsible for 3.4 million deaths worldwide. In 1980, an estimated 28.8% of men and 29.8% of women worldwide had a body mass index of 25 kg/m$^2$ or greater, while in 2013 these percentages had risen to 36.9% of men and 38% of women (see Table 1). The highest prevalence of obesity (>50%) was identified in Tonga, Kuwait, Libya, Qatar, and Samoa, while the lowest prevalence of obesity was reported from Vietnam. Of importance, there was no nation demonstrating any apparent improvement over the past 33 years. Morbid obesity has been directly associated with significant co-morbid conditions, including the metabolic syndrome, obstructive sleep apnea, certain carcinomas, and non-alcoholic steatohepatitis.

Due to poor results involving maintenance therapy, weight loss through specific lifestyle modifications including diet and exercise are generally ineffective for producing sustained weight loss.

## Surgical Treatment of Obesity

Because of insufficient results obtained with diet and activity programs, bariatric surgery has become an important option for individuals with medically-complicated obesity. In the United States, the most common bariatric surgical procedure is yet Roux-en-Y gastric bypass.

**Table 1. Definition of Obesity by BMI* and the Worldwide Prevalence of Overweight/Obesity**

| BMI* | YEAR (SEX) | DEFINITION | OBESITY CLASS | WORLDWIDE BMI >24.9 |
|---|---|---|---|---|
| 18.5-24.9 | | Normal | | |
| 25-29.9 | | Overweight | | |
| 30-34.9 | | Obesity | I | |
| 35-39.9 | | Obesity | II | |
| >39.9 | | Obesity | III | |
| | 1980<br>FEMALES<br>MALES | | | <br>29.8%<br>28.8% |
| | 2013<br>FEMALES<br>MALES | | | <br>38%<br>36.9 |

*BMI = Body Mass Index in kg/m$^2$.

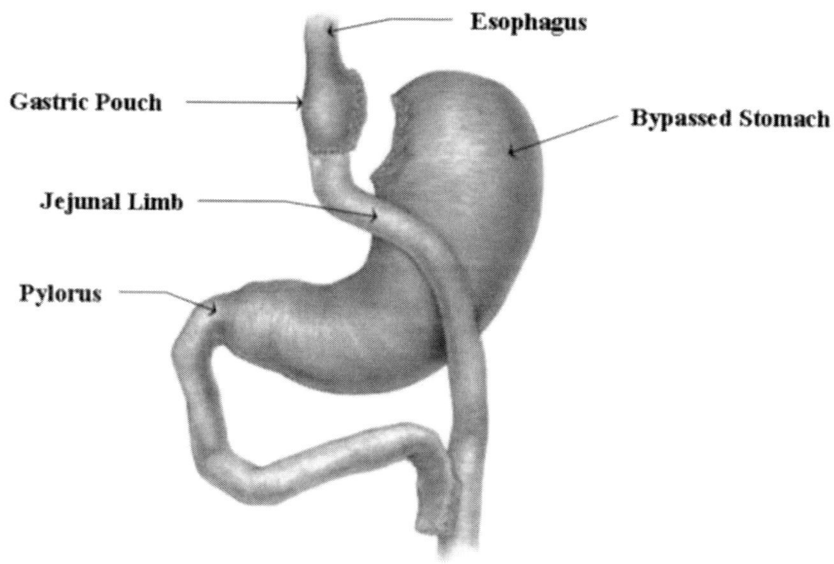


Figure 1. Roux-en-Y Gastric Bypass Surgery. Intestinal digestion and absorption is in continuity with the jejunal limb. The length of the pancreatico-biliary limb is represented by the distance from the pylorus to the jejuno-jejunal anastomosis and is the bypassed small intestine. Small intestine distal to the jejuno-jejunal anastomosis (the common channel) permits mixing of micronutrients (including Vitamin D) with bile. A longer pancreatico-biliary limb decreases the surface area of small intestine available for the absorption of micronutrients (Reproduced with permission from Lakhani, SV; et al. *Nutrition Res* 2008; 28(5): 293-298.).

As shown in Figure 1, this procedure involves both complete division of the upper stomach and transection of the small intestine approximately 75 cm distal to the ligament of Treitz.

This leaves an upper pouch of stomach with a volume of 15 to 30 milliliters which is connected (the gastrojejunal anastomosis) to the distal segment of transected jejunum, while the proximal segment of transected jejunum is anastomosed to jejunum approximately 100 cm distal to the gastrojejunal anastomosis. Intestinal digestion and absorption is in continuity with the jejunal limb. The length of the pancreatico-biliary limb is represented by the distance from the pylorus to the jejuno-jejunal anastomosis and is the bypassed small intestine. Small intestine distal to the jejuno-jejunal anastomosis (the common channel) permits mixing of micronutrients (including Vitamin D) with bile. A longer pancreatico-biliary limb decreases the surface area of small intestine available for the absorption of micronutrients. A shorter common channel to the ileocecal valve can result in decreased absorption involving bile acids, which includes absorption of vitamin D, a fat soluble vitamin. Creation of a shorter common channel may also alter motility and possibly the bacterial flora or microbiota of the upper intestinal tract.

Bariatric surgical procedures are considered by individuals with a body mass index >39.9 $kg/m^2$, or body mass index of >34.9 $kg/m^2$ with an associated significant co-morbidity. Clinical outcome studies have shown significant resolution of hypertension, hyperlipidemia, and diabetes mellitus in patients after Roux-en-Y gastric bypass [2]. Studies have also shown significant reductions in long-term mortality after gastric bypass surgery, and this included mortality induced by cardiovascular events, diabetes, and cancer [3, 4]. These outcome studies support the utilization of bariatric surgery for the treatment of medically-complicated obesity.

The types of bariatric procedures performed can alter the rates of nutritional deficiencies. Bariatric procedures may involve surgery on the stomach, or surgery on the stomach and small intestine (such as divided Roux-en-Y gastric bypass). Bariatric surgeries on the stomach are in general restrictive, while surgery on the small intestine may induce additional malabsorption. Bariatric procedures designed to have a malabsorptive component often produce greater nutritional deficiencies than restrictive strategies.

An adjustable gastric band is primarily a restrictive strategy that does not bypass any part of the GI tract and there is no reduction in the capacity of the stomach. At laparoscopy, a plastic latch is used to hold a soft, silicone ring circumferentially around the upper stomach about 4 cm distal to the gastroesophageal junction. A subcutaneous access port is connected via tubing the silicone ring or band. Sterile fluid added to the port induces extrinsic restriction of the upper stomach lumen by the silicone ring.

Vertical sleeve gastrectomy is another primarily restrictive procedure which involves reduction of the stomach size. The surgical construction of a vertical sleeve gastrectomy involves resection of 60% to 80% of the stomach along the greater curvature by using multiple staplers to produce a tubular gastric pouch.

Vertical-banded gastroplasty is another restrictive strategy that involves creation of a small stomach pouch through a combination of banding (a non-adjustable band in the upper stomach) and stapling of the body of the stomach; this procedure is now rarely performed [5].

# Overview of the Physiology of Vitamin D

Vitamin D is one of the four major fat-soluble vitamins. Vitamin D is involved in the regulation of multiple physiological processes in the body including mood, inflammation, immunity, and bone health. It has been shown that Vitamin D3 in human skin is produced by conversion of 7-dehydrocholesterol during exposure to sunlight [6]. Accumulation of Vitamin D3 is limited to 10-15% of the tissue 7-dehydrocholesterol. Seven days after total body exposure to ultraviolet radiation, serum 25-hydroxyvitamin D levels increase. However, individuals may not have adequate sun exposure, and therefore require dietary intake of vitamin D. The absorption of vitamin D is a complex process that takes place in the small intestine and is influenced by pancreatic secretion, bile, and integrity of the intestinal wall.

Earlier work in this field had shown that the principal storage sites of Vitamin D in humans are adipose tissue and striated muscle [7]. Produced 25-hydroxyvitamin D is taken up from the blood into many tissues in humans. Vitamin D can be excreted into the bile. A more recent study in humans has confirmed the storage of Vitamin D in fat tissue samples [8]. Indeed, there was a positive correlation between Vitamin D3 levels in fat tissue and in serum samples. This finding supports fat tissue as a storage site for Vitamin D and supports serum Vitamin D3 levels as a reflection of total Vitamin D3 stores in humans.

Vitamin D is an important factor in calcium regulation and is involved in prevention of hypocalcemia, secondary hyperparathyroidism, osteoporosis, and osteomalacia. Vitamin D regulates skeletal calcium balance by increasing calcium absorption by the intestine. Vitamin D assists in the maintenance of adequate calcium and phosphate levels required for bone formation thereby allowing proper functioning of the parathyroid hormone [9].

In individuals with inadequate vitamin D stores, there is inadequate calcium absorption and utilization. Hypocalcemia can lead to release of calcium stores as the results of feedback from increased release of parathyroid hormone and increased calcium reabsorption from the bones, with secondary decreased urinary calcium secretion [10]. Vitamin D deficiency is therefore important in the activation of a metabolic cascade that results in bone loss and can increase the risk of developing bone fractures.

# Vitamin D and Obesity

There are several observational studies that have examined Vitamin D in individuals with obesity. There has been an examination of Vitamin D in the National Health and Nutrition Examination Survey 1988 to 1994 [11]. Vitamin D serum levels were decreased in obese women. There has also been an examination of Vitamin D in the National Health and Nutrition Examination Survey 2005 to 2006 [12]. In this study, Vitamin D deficiency was defined by a serum 25-hydroxyvitamin D level of <20 ng/ml or 50 nmol/L. The global prevalence of Vitamin D deficiency in this survey was 41.6%, with the highest rates identified in black Americans at 82.1%. Vitamin D deficiency was significantly more common in obese individuals. An absence of daily milk consumption was independently associated with Vitamin D deficiency.

Preoperative determination of Vitamin D levels in obese individuals considering bariatric surgery has identified similar findings. In a study of 379 preoperative bariatric patients,

Vitamin D deficiency was present in 68% of these individuals [13]. In a recent study of 115 women considering bariatric surgery, 71.3% had Vitamin D deficiency [14]. However, these preoperative surveys did not provide information about the mechanisms of Vitamin D deficiency in obese individuals.

## Vitamin D and Bariatric Surgery

Older studies had supported the importance of the stomach in the prevention of Vitamin D deficiency. In a study of 25 individuals who had undergone total gastrectomy, serum 25-hydroxyvitamin D levels were significantly decreased post-operatively [15]. These findings were associated with increased serum alkaline phosphatase levels and increased urinary excretion of cyclic AMP. It was suggested that in individuals after total gastrectomy, there is defective Vitamin D storage and enhanced Vitamin D action as a compensatory mechanism induced by sustained calcium deficiency.

Despite the promising results in sustained weight loss after bariatric surgical procedures, chronic complications including macronutrient and micronutrient deficiencies can develop. Micronutrient disorders including vitamin D deficiency are commonly found in individuals before bariatric surgery and have been shown to persist after bariatric surgery. Vitamin D deficiency is a major clinical concern since bariatric patients are at risk for developing osteoporosis and osteomalacia.

There have been multiple studies of Vitamin D deficiency after bariatric surgery (see Table 2). There are wide variations reported in the post-operative prevalence of Vitamin D deficiency likely due to the type of hospital involved in bariatric surgery and the length of follow-up. In a study from a University Hospital [16], 318 individuals had serum Vitamin D levels examined at 1 year after surgery. In this study the prevalence of Vitamin D deficiency was 7%. In a more recent study [17], 293 individuals (83% females) had serum Vitamin D levels measured a mean of 11 years after Roux-en-Y gastric bypass. The prevalence of Vitamin D deficiency in this long term study was 65%. Multiple studies have documented the potential of Roux-en-Y gastric bypass to cause bone loss as the result of vitamin D deficiency.

Despite the potential minimization of malabsorption in individuals undergoing vertical sleeve gastrectomy, there is emerging scientific literature that Vitamin D deficiency is common after sleeve gastrectomy. This is important due to the worldwide rise in the utilization of vertical sleeve gastrectomy. In 2008, only 4% of bariatric surgical procedures were a vertical sleeve gastrectomy, but this had risen to 19% by 2011 [18]. There has been short term as well as long term studies of the prevalence of Vitamin D deficiency after vertical sleeve gastrectomy that has been published.

In a one year follow up of 60 individuals after vertical sleeve gastrectomy, Aarts et al reported a 39% prevalence of Vitamin D deficiency [19]. In a second one year follow up of 64 individuals after vertical sleeve gastrectomy, Toh and associates [20] reported a 43% prevalence of Vitamin D deficiency. The results for long term follow up studies are similar. At 5 years after vertical sleeve gastrectomy, Saif et al reported a 42% prevalence of Vitamin D deficiency [21]. Within 3 years after vertical sleeve gastrectomy, Gehrer and associates

**Table 2. Prevalence of Vitamin D Deficiency After Bariatric Surgery**

| SURGERY* | POST-OPERATIVE TIME PERIOD | NUMBER OF PATIENTS | VITAMIN D DEFICIENCY | REFERENCE |
|---|---|---|---|---|
| RYGB | 1 Year | 318 | 7% | 16 |
| RYGB | 11 Years | 293 | 65% | 17 |
| VSG | 1 Year | 60 | 39% | 19 |
| VSG | 1 Year | 64 | 43% | 20 |
| VSG | 5 Years | 30 | 42% | 21 |
| VSG | 3 Years | 50 | 32% | 22 |
| VSG | 4 Years | 61 | 37% | 23 |
| AGB | 1 Year | 50 | 8% | 24 |
| AGB | 1 Year | 17 | 41% | 25 |

*RYGB: Roux-en-Y Gastric Bypass; VSG: Vertical Sleeve Gastrectomy;
AGB: Adjustable Gastric Band.

[22] found a 32% prevalence of Vitamin D deficiency. These results have been confirmed by an additional 4 year study that confirmed a 37% prevalence of Vitamin D deficiency after vertical sleeve gastrectomy [23].

By contrast to vertical sleeve gastrectomy, the worldwide performance of adjustable gastric banding has fallen from 44% of bariatric surgical procedures in 2008 to 27% in 2011 [18]. In individuals who have undergone laparoscopic adjustable gastric banding, a study of adolescents revealed Vitamin D deficiency to be the second most common micronutrient deficiency within the first two years after surgery [24]. In a 1 year follow up after performing adjustable gastric banding, Fish and associates [25] reported continued Vitamin D deficiency in 41% of individuals.

It has been suggested that patients who have undergone a gastric restrictive procedure such as vertical sleeve gastrectomy or adjustable gastric banding have significantly higher Vitamin D levels and improvement in Vitamin D deficiency. The published results do not strongly support this notion. Gehrer et at [22] reported 2 years post-operatively that 28% of individuals who had undergone sleeve gastrectomy were Vitamin D deficient while 47% of individuals who had undergone Roux-en-Y gastric bypass were Vitamin D deficient. By contrast, Moize and associates have reported that at 4-5 years post-operatively the prevalence of Vitamin D deficiency is 37% in individuals who had undergone vertical sleeve gastrectomy and 32.5% in individuals who had undergone Roux-en-Y gastric bypass. An additional study suggested initial improvement in serum 25-hydroxy Vitamin D levels after adjustable gastric banding compared to Roux-en-Y gastric bypass [26]. However, the improvements in serum vitamin D levels declined over an 18 month period, while changes in levels of parathyroid hormone supported increased bone turnover. These results do not support the idea that bypassing small intestine significantly increases the post-operative risk of Vitamin D deficiency.

Vitamin D deficiency after bariatric surgery induces inadequate calcium absorption and utilization [27, 28]. As a result of a hypocalcemic state, calcium stores can be mobilized by feedback activation of the parathyroid glands. Studies have shown that the prevalence of secondary hyperparathyroidism may reach 58% in individuals after Roux-en-Y gastric bypass surgery [17]. Subsequently, osteoporosis and osteomalacia may develop increasing the risk of any fracture after Roux-en-Y gastric bypass by 2.3-fold [29].

An increased risk of bone disease has in addition been reported in individuals after vertical sleeve gastrectomy [30]. The authors report results from 29 women with a mean age of 41.1 years. In this group, 87% of the women were premenopausal. After vertical sleeve gastrectomy, these individuals lost a mean of 46.5% of their excess body weight at 6 months. Bone density studies revealed that at baseline, two women (7%) had evidence for low bone mass, while at 6 month follow-up, two women (7%) still had low bone mass and two additional women (7%) developed T-scores suggesting low bone mass. These studies support the concern that Vitamin D deficiency after both Roux-en-Y gastric bypass and vertical sleeve gastrectomy can lead to bone disease.

## Proposed Mechanisms of Vitamin D Deficiency after Bariatric Surgery

Despite multiple publications describing this condition and its outcome, the underlying mechanisms involved in the development of Vitamin D deficiency post operatively are not well understood. As shown in Table 3, many mechanisms have been proposed as to why Vitamin D deficiency is so prevalent after bariatric surgery. Deficiency of Vitamin D may occur after bariatric surgical procedures as the result of gastric reduction, decreased intake of nutrient-rich foods, poor food tolerability, and noncompliance with Vitamin D supplementation. Patients may experience vomiting after bariatric procedures, which puts them at risk for decreased nutritional intake. Other complications including diarrhea from fat malabsorption and dumping syndrome may also result in vitamin D deficiency [31].

Published studies have suggested that bariatric surgical procedures which utilize restrictive strategies may initially improve vitamin D deficiency compared to bariatric procedures which utilize both restriction and malabsorption.

As we describe, long term follow up of vertical sleeve gastrectomy and Roux-en-Y gastric bypass reveal that Vitamin D deficiency is similar for both procedures. Therefore, the question arises as to why there is a high prevalence of Vitamin D deficiency even after a restrictive procedure such as sleeve gastrectomy. These results support the suggestion that another mechanism is responsible for post-operative vitamin D deficiency.

**Table 3. Proposed Mechanisms for Development of Vitamin D Deficiency After Bariatric Surgery**

| |
|---|
| Gastric Reduction |
| Noncompliance with Vitamin D Supplementation |
| Inadequate Dietary Intake of Vitamin D |
| - Decreased Intake of Nutrient-Rich Foods |
| - Poor Food Tolerability |
| - Post-Operative Vomiting |
| Altered Intestinal Absorption or Storage of Vitamin D in Obesity |
| Bile Acid Deficiency |
| Dumping Syndrome with Rapid Oral-Cecal Transit |
| Utilization During the Rapid Weight Loss Phase |
| Small Intestinal Bacterial Overgrowth |

## Vitamin D Deficiency and Small Intestinal Bacterial Overgrowth

A clinical diagnosis of small intestinal bacterial overgrowth can be difficult since patients can present after bariatric surgery with non-specific symptoms including cramping abdominal pain, abdominal bloating or distension, increased flatulence, or diarrhea. These symptoms can overlap with symptoms of malabsorption due to lactose intolerance or surgical bypass of small intestine.

Small intestinal bacterial overgrowth after gastrointestinal surgery has long been known to lead to Vitamin B12 deficiency, and our group has more recently described the role of small intestinal bacterial overgrowth in development of Vitamin B1 deficiency [32]. The results of our studies suggested that small intestinal bacterial overgrowth is a potential mechanism to explain post-operative micronutrient deficiencies.

Our studies have also expanded upon prior reports of increased serum levels of folate (produced by upper intestinal bacteria) in individuals with small intestinal bacterial overgrowth [33]. This syndrome results in malabsorption as the result of alterations in the microbiota of the gastrointestinal tract. In normal healthy individuals, there are low concentrations of colonization of bacteria in the proximal gastrointestinal tract. However in small intestinal bacterial overgrowth, the flora of the proximal small intestine is changed to higher concentrations of anaerobic bacteria that can induce fermentation.

Bariatric surgery can impair the normal defenses against bacterial overgrowth in the upper gastrointestinal tract. These physiologic defenses include stomach acid, gastric emptying, intraluminal bile acids, pancreatic enzymes, the intestinal immune system, and small intestinal motility (the inter-digestive migrating motor complex). Small intestinal motility and the migrating motor complex are important defense mechanisms against SIBO likely due to passage of bacteria into the colon [34]. Bariatric surgery can disrupt these defense mechanisms. The creation of a short common channel results in less time and less intestinal surface area for bile acids, gastric acids, and pancreatic enzymes to digest and limit bacterial overgrowth. Roux-en-Y gastric bypass surgery produces a blind limb between the bypassed stomach and the jejuno-jejunal anastomosis (see Figure 1). Post-procedural disruptions that impair small intestinal motility, including medications, also allow bacteria to have prolonged access to intestinal chyme and appear to promote small intestinal bacterial overgrowth [35].

Therefore, based upon prior reports of B vitamin deficiencies induced by small intestinal bacterial overgrowth, our group examined the association between calcium metabolism and small intestinal bacterial overgrowth [36]. This study was a retrospective, observational evaluation of 452 patients who underwent Roux-en-Y gastric bypass surgery at our institution from 1999 to 2005. All patients at our institution are instructed to take by mouth 1.0 gram daily of calcium and 2 chewable multivitamins daily containing 800 Units (20 mcg) of Vitamin D. Patients taking diuretics were excluded from the study. Levels of serum folate, serum calcium, and 24 hour urinary calcium levels were available in 154 of these gastric bypass patients. An elevated serum folate level was accepted as a level that was above the upper limit of normal for the serum folate assay. Glucose-hydrogen breath testing was performed in 44 patients (an abnormal glucose-hydrogen breath test was defined by: hydrogen concentration rising >15 parts per million over the baseline fasting value or a fasting hydrogen level >10 parts per million). Corrected serum calcium levels were within normal limits in all patients in this study. This finding is consistent with reports from other groups that serum calcium is a poor determinant of calcium metabolism after bariatric surgery.

**Table 4. Sensitivity (38/42 = 90%) of Elevated Serum Folate As a Surrogate Marker for Small Intestinal Bacterial Overgrowth (Chi-Squared 2x2: P < .001)**

| | Normal Folate | Elevated Folate | Total |
|---|---|---|---|
| Normal Glucose-H2 Breath Test | 2 | 0 | 2 |
| Abnormal Glucose-H2 Breath Test | 4 | 38 | 42 |
| Total | 6 | 38 | 44 |

In our results, as shown in Table 4, of the 42 individuals with an abnormal glucose-hydrogen breath test consistent with a diagnosis of small intestinal bacterial overgrowth, 38 individuals also had an elevated serum folate level. This finding supported a sensitivity of 90% (38/42) for the use of elevated serum folate level as a surrogate marker for small intestinal bacterial overgrowth (Chi-squared 2X2: p < .001).

The potential role of small intestinal bacterial overgrowth in the alteration of calcium metabolism after Roux-en-Y gastric bypass was supported by two additional results.

As shown in Table 5, there were 42 individuals with an abnormal glucose-hydrogen breath test supporting a diagnosis of small intestinal bacterial overgrowth. Of these 42 individuals, 30 were found to have low 24 hour urinary calcium levels (Chi-squared 2x2: p<.01), supporting the presence of calcium deficiency in individuals with small intestinal bacterial overgrowth.

**Table 5. Relationship between Abnormal Glucose-Hydrogen Breath Testing And Calcium Deficiency (Chi-Squared 2x2: P < .001)**

| | Normal Urinary Calcium | Low Urinary Calcium | Total |
|---|---|---|---|
| Normal Glucose Hydrogen Breath Test | 8 | 3 | 11 |
| Abnormal Glucose Hydrogen Breath Test | 1 | 30 | 31 |
| Total | 9 | 33 | 42 |

As shown in Table 6, there were 106 individuals with elevated serum folate levels, supporting a diagnosis of small intestinal bacterial overgrowth. Of these 106 individuals, 80 patients had low 24 hour urinary calcium levels (Chi-squared 2x2: p<.001), supporting the presence of calcium deficiency in individuals with small intestinal bacterial overgrowth.

**Table 6. Relationship between Elevated Serum Folate Levels and Calcium Deficiency (Chi Squared 2X2: p< .001)**

| | Normal Urinary Calcium | Low Urinary Calcium | Total |
|---|---|---|---|
| Normal Folate | 38 | 10 | 48 |
| Elevated Folate | 26 | 80 | 106 |
| Total | 64 | 90 | 154 |

These results supported our hypothesis that patients who undergo bariatric surgery may be at risk for developing calcium deficiency due to the effect of small intestinal bacterial overgrowth on Vitamin D metabolism. In previous studies, our group has shown that treatment of Vitamin B1 deficiency with oral Vitamin B1 supplements requires concomitant antibiotic therapy for small intestinal bacterial overgrowth [32]. This finding suggests that oral Vitamin D supplements may not be fully effective for the treatment of Vitamin D deficiency in individuals who have small intestinal bacterial overgrowth after bariatric surgery. The question of how Vitamin D malabsorption may be induced by small intestinal bacterial overgrowth requires further evaluation through a translational research study. A clinical trial could be developed to evaluate treatment of small intestinal bacterial overgrowth and the subsequent absorption of oral Vitamin D.

## Screening for Vitamin D Deficiency

Physicians should be aware of the risk of Vitamin D deficiency and the need to monitor bariatric patients closely. Regular follow-up can be important for preventing the development of Vitamin D deficiency and its sequelae in this susceptible group. Patients who undergo bariatric surgery may maintain normal serum calcium concentrations by increasing the release of calcium from bone and decreasing urinary calcium secretion. Therefore, isolated measurements of serum calcium concentrations are not adequate markers of calcium metabolism in these patients post-operatively.

The clinical presentation of Vitamin D deficiency can include depression, bony pain, low back pain, aching of the limbs, or a chronic pain syndrome. Altered calcium metabolism is supported by a decreased 24 hour urinary calcium levels, but this result can be altered by concomitant use of diuretics.

Routine screening for nutrient deficiencies is recommended in obese patients pre-operatively and post-operatively following bariatric surgery, because these patients have an increased risk for deficiencies [37]. The 2013 joint guidelines from the American Association of Clinical Endocrinologists, The Obesity Society, and the American Society for Metabolic and Bariatric Surgery recommend pre-operative nutrient screening which includes a 25-hydroxy Vitamin D level. The joint guidelines recommend more extensive testing in those individuals undergoing malabsorptive bariatric procedures.

For monitoring purposes, a 24 hour urinary calcium level and serum alkaline phosphatase measurement every 6 to 12 months has been suggested after Roux-en-Y gastric bypass [38]. Based on the high prevalence of Vitamin D deficiency after vertical sleeve gastrectomy, active screening of these bariatric patients should also be considered. If the urine calcium excretion is low and the serum alkaline phosphatase activity is increased, alkaline phosphatase can be fractionated or a serum parathyroid level should be ordered. If the alkaline phosphatase elevation is of bone origin, the serum parathyroid hormone level should certainly be measured. Elevated serum parathyroid levels require aggressive supplementation with both Vitamin D and calcium, and ongoing surveillance. A total 25-hydroxy Vitamin D level should be considered every 12 months after malabsorptive bariatric surgery, or sooner if a patient has a low 24 hour urinary calcium excretion. A bone density scan to assess the individual for bone loss should be considered in those patients who have not had regular follow-up following bariatric surgery and who present with clinical and biochemical evidence for Vitamin D deficiency.

## Management of Vitamin D Deficiency after Bariatric Surgery

As described in our above sections, there is a high prevalence of Vitamin D deficiency after both Roux-en-Y gastric bypass and vertical sleeve gastrectomy. Current clinical guidelines recommend daily oral Vitamin D supplementation after bariatric surgery. However, the high rates of persistent vitamin D deficiency are concerning.

Post-operatively, it is now recommended that all individuals who have undergone Roux-en-Y gastric bypass or vertical sleeve gastrectomy receive daily micronutrient supplementation consisting of two multivitamin supplements (to include iron, folic acid, thiamine, and Vitamin B12), 1500 mg of elemental calcium, and at least 3000 international units or 75 mcg of vitamin D (titrated to maintain serum 25-hydroxy Vitamin D levels >30 ng/ml) for minimally the first 3 to 6 months after surgery [37]. Many health care professionals prescribe Vitamin D3 (cholecalciferol) more frequently than Vitamin D2 (ergocalciferol) as the preferred form of oral Vitamin D supplementation.

The recommended "optimal" dose of oral vitamin D supplementation for individuals who have undergone bariatric surgery has varied in the available literature. The post-operative joint recommendations were revised recently [37] with the suggestion of an increase to 3000 international units of Vitamin D supplementation daily. Prior to this update, recommendations following bariatric surgery ranged from 800 international units to 50,000 international units per day of Vitamin D, depending upon the individual's requirements. These recommendations are much higher than the Institute of Medicine's recommended dietary allowances of 600 international units per day in non-operative adults who are 19 to 70 years-old [39].

A recent prospective study was designed to clarify the optimal levels of supplementation of Vitamin D among different bariatric surgical procedures [40]. Vitamin D and calcium levels were measured in women who received 2,000 international units of Vitamin D3 and 1,500 mg calcium citrate daily for 3 months after either Roux-en-Y gastric bypass or sleeve gastrectomy. Patients' height, weight, body mass index, serum 25-hydroxy Vitamin D, and serum parathyroid concentrations were measured preoperatively and at 3 months post-operatively. The investigators reported that Vitamin D deficiency decreased from 60.6% preoperatively to 26.1% after 3 months ($P<0.005$), that serum 25-hydroxy Vitamin D concentrations increased an average of 8 ng/mL ($P<0.001$), and that parathyroid hormone concentrations decreased an average of 9 ng/L (this reduction was not significant). Interestingly, this study revealed no difference overall in the response to supplementation following Roux-en-Y gastric bypass or vertical sleeve gastrectomy. The study did support the 2013 guidelines for higher amounts of Vitamin D3 supplementation following bariatric surgery [37].

In those patients who have low serum levels of 25-hydroxyvitamin D, it is suggested that the individual begin 50,000 international units (1250 mcg) of vitamin D (ergocalciferol) orally taken once per week for 6 to 8 weeks. This treatment is followed up with a repeat 25-hydroxyvitamin D level after 8 weeks in order to evaluate repletion of Vitamin D [41].

Al-Shoha et al have reported five patients after gastric bypass surgery with bone biopsy-proven osteomalacia and bone marrow fibrosis [42]. These five patients had reported symptoms for 2 to 5 years. Treatment included a combination of ergocalciferol (100,000 international units or 2500 mcg daily) and calcium carbonate (1 to 2.5 g daily). The authors did report that there was significant improvement in the patients' clinical symptoms, functional status, biochemical indices, and bone mineral density after initiation of treatment.

## Conclusion

As the prevalence of obesity and its comorbid conditions continue to increase, bariatric surgical procedures remain a major option for the treatment of medically-complicated obesity. These bariatric surgical procedures are not without consequences and nutritional deficiencies including Vitamin D deficiency remain as significant clinical concerns. Bariatric patients who have Vitamin D deficiency are at risk for developing osteoporosis and osteomalacia, especially if there has been insufficient screening for and treatment of Vitamin D deficiency, both pre-operatively and long-term post-operatively. Despite prescribing Vitamin D oral supplementation after bariatric surgical procedures, the rates of vitamin D deficiency post-operatively remain high. Bariatric surgical procedures that include a restrictive component with less malabsorptive component may develop lower rates of Vitamin D deficiency in the short term period, as the result of improvements in Vitamin D deficiency after supplementation. However, long term follow up of these patients show that another mechanism may be important for the persistence of Vitamin D deficiency despite the use of oral Vitamin D supplementation. Our studies support the concern that small intestinal bacterial overgrowth may induce malabsorption of oral Vitamin D. This is the potential mechanism for the persistent Vitamin D deficiency in patients after bariatric surgery who are receiving oral Vitamin D supplementation. Clinicians should maintain increased suspicion for the presence of small intestinal bacterial overgrowth in those patients with persistent vitamin D deficiency following bariatric surgery.

Recommendations for the adequate supplementation of oral Vitamin D after bariatric surgery have varied and have only recently begun to address the problem of persistent vitamin D deficiency by increasing the recommended amount of daily oral Vitamin D to 3000 international units (75 mcg).

Improved understanding of the mechanisms involved in pre-operative Vitamin D deficiency and the disorders that inhibit repletion of Vitamin D after bariatric surgery are important in order to improve the treatment of Vitamin D deficiency in individuals who undergo bariatric surgery. Future studies should demonstrate a reduction in the risks of developing osteoporosis and osteomalacia in those bariatric patients who improve their repletion of Vitamin D.

## References

[1] Ng, M; Fleming, T; Robinson, M; et al. Global, regional and national prevalence of overweight and obesity in children and adults during 1980-2013: A systematic analysis for the Global Burden of Disease Study 2013. *Lancet* 2014; 384(9945):766-81.

[2] Adams, TD; Pendleton, RC; Strong, MB; et al. Health outcomes of gastric bypass patients compared to nonsurgical, nonintervened severely obese. *Obesity (Silver Spring)* 2010; 18(1): 121-30.

[3] Sjöström, L; Narbro, K; Sjöström, CD. Effects of bariatric surgery on mortality in Swedish obese subjects. *N Engl J Med* 2007; 357(8): 741-52.

[4] Adams, TD; Gress, RE; Smith, SC. Long-term mortality after gastric bypass surgery. *N Engl J Med* 2007; 357(8): 753-61.

[5] Bal, BS; Finelli, FC; Shope, TR; Koch, TR. Nutritional deficiencies after bariatric surgery. *Nat Rev Endocrinol* 2012; 8: 544–56.

[6] Holick, MF. The cutaneous photosynthesis of previtamin D3: a unique photoendocrine system. *J Invest Dermatol* 1981; 77: 51-8.

[7] Mawer, EB; Backhouse, J; Holman, CA; Lumb, GA; Stanbury, SW. The distribution and storage of vitamin D and its metabolites in human tissues. Clin Sci 1972; 43: 413-31.

[8] Blum, M; Dolnikowski, G; Seyoum, E; Harris, SS; Booth, SL; Peterson, J; Saltzman, E; Dawson-Hughes, B. Vitamin D(3) in fat tissue. Endocrine 2008; 33: 90-4.

[9] Bell, TD; Demay, MB; Burnett-Bowie, SAM. The biology and pathology of vitamin D control in bone. *J Cell Biochem* 2010; 111 (1): 7–13.

[10] Eliel, LP; Chanes, R; Hawrylko, J. Influence of parathyroid activity on ion exchange in various tissues. *Trans Am Clin Climatol Assoc* 1962; 74: 130-8.

[11] Kimmons, JE; Blanck, HM; Tohill, BC; Zhang, J; Khan, LK. Associations between body mass index and the prevalence of low micronutrient levels among US adults. *Med Gen Med* 2006; 8(4): 59.

[12] Forrest, KYZ; Stuhldreher, WL. Prevalence and correlates of vitamin D deficiency in US adults. *Nutrition Res* 2011; 31: 48-54.

[13] Flancbaum, L; Belsley, S; Drake, V; Colarusso, T; Tayler, E. Preoperative nutritional status of patients undergoing Roux-en-Y gastric bypass for morbid obesity. *J Gastrointest Surg* 2006; 10: 1033-7.

[14] de Luis, DA; Pacheco, D; Izaola, O; Terroba, MC; Cuellar, L; Cabezas, G. Micronutrient status in morbidly obese women before bariatric surgery. *Surg Obes Relat Dis* 2013; 9: 323-7.

[15] Kozawa, K; Imawari, M; Shimazu, H; Kobori, O; Osuga, T; Morioka, Y. Vitamin D status after total gastrectomy. *Dig Dis Sci* 1984; 29: 411-6.

[16] Clements, RH; Katasani, VG; Palepu, R; et al. Incidence of vitamin deficiency after laparoscopic Roux-en-Y gastric bypass in a university hospital setting. *Am Surg* 2006; 72(12): 1196-202.

[17] Karefylakis, C; Näslund, I; Edholm, D; Sundbom, M; Karlsson, FA; Rask, E. Vitamin D status 10 years after primary gastric bypass: Gravely high prevalence of hypovitaminosis D and raised PTH levels. *Obes Surg* 2014; 24(3): 343-8.

[18] Buchwald, H; Oien, DM. Metabolic/bariatric surgery worldwide 2011. *Obes Surg* 2013; 23: 427-36.

[19] Aarts, EO; Janssen, IM; Berends, FJ. The gastric sleeve: Losing weight as fast as micronutrients? *Obes Surg* 2011; 21: 207-11.

[20] Toh, SY; Zarshenas, N; Jorgensen, J. Prevalence of nutrient deficiencies in bariatric patients. *Nutrition* 2009; 25: 1150-6.

[21] Saif, T; Strain, GW; Dakin, G; Gagner, M; Costa, R; Pomp, A. Evaluation of nutrient status after laparoscopic sleeve gastrectomy 1, 3, and 5 years after surgery. *Surg Obes Relat Dis* 2012; 8: 542-7.

[22] Gehrer, S; Kern, B; Peters, T; Christoffel-Courtin, C; Peterli, R. Fewer nutrient deficiencies after laparoscopic sleeve gastrectomy (LSG) than after laparoscopic Roux-Y-gastric bypass (LRYGB)-a prospective study. *Obes Surg* 2010; 20: 447-53.

[23] Moizé, V; Andreu, A; Flores, L; Torres, F; Ibarzabal, A; Delgado, S; Lacy, A; Rodriguez, L; Vidal, J. Long-term dietary intake and nutritional deficiencies following

sleeve gastrectomy or Roux-En-Y gastric bypass in a mediterranean population. *J Acad Nutr Diet* 2013; 113: 400-10.
[24] Nadler, EP; Youn, HA; Ren, CJ; Fielding, GA. An update on 73 US obese pediatric patients treated with laparoscopic adjustable gastric banding: comorbidity resolution and compliance data. *J Pediatr Surg* 2008; 43: 141-6.
[25] Fish, E; Beverstein, G; Olson, D; Reinhardt, S; Garren, M; Gould, J. Vitamin D status of morbidly obese bariatric surgery patients. *J Surg Res* 2010; 164: 198-202.
[26] Sinha, N; Shieh, A; Stein, EM; et al. Increased PTH and 1.25(OH)(2)D levels associated with increased markers of bone turnover following bariatric surgery. *Obesity (Silver Spring)* 2011; 19(12): 2388-93.
[27] El-Kadre, LJ; Rocha, PRS; de Almeida Tinoco, AC; Tinoco, RC. Calcium metabolism in pre- and postmenopausal morbidly obese women at baseline and after laparoscopic Roux-en-Y gastric bypass. *Obesity Surg* 2004; 14: 1062-1066.
[28] Youssef, Y; Richards, WO; Sekhar, N; Kaiser, J; Spagnoli, A; Abumrad, N; et al. Risk of secondary hyperparathyroidism after laparoscopic gastric bypass surgery in obese women. *Surg Endosc* 2007; 21(8): 1393-6.
[29] Nakamura, KM; Haglind, EG; Clowes, JA; Achenbach, SJ; Atkinson, EJ; Melton, LJ 3rd; Kennel, KA. Fracture risk following bariatric surgery: A population-based study. *Osteoporos Int* 2014; 25: 151-8.
[30] Pluskiewicz, W; Bužga, M; Holéczy, P; Bortlík, L; Šmajstrla, V; Adamczyk, P. Bone mineral changes in spine and proximal femur in individual obese women after laparoscopic sleeve gastrectomy: a short-term study. *Obes Surg* 2012; 22: 1068-76.
[31] Levinson, R; Silverman, JB; Catella, JG; et al. Pharmacotherapy prevention and management of nutritional deficiencies post Roux-en-Y gastric bypass. *Obes Surg* 2013; 23(7): 992-1000.
[32] Lakhani, SV; Shah, HN; Alexander, K; FC; Kirkpatrick, JR; Koch, TR. Small intestinal bacterial overgrowth and thiamine deficiency after Roux-en-Y gastric bypass surgery in obese patients. *Nutrition Res* 2008; 28(5): 293-298.
[33] Camilo, E; Zimmerman, J; Mason, JB; et al. Folate synthesized by bacteria in the human upper small intestine is assimilated by the host. *Gastroenterology* 1996; 110(4): 991-8.
[34] Singh, VV; Toskes, PP. Small bowel bacterial overgrowth: Presentation, diagnosis, and treatment. *Curr Gastro Rep* 2003; 5: 365-372.
[35] Bal, BS; Shah, HN; Finelli, FC; Kirkpatrick, JR; Koch, TR. Risk factors associated with small intestinal bacterial overgrowth after Roux-en-Y gastric bypass surgery. *Am J Gastroenterol* 2008; 103(S1): S97-8.
[36] Bal, BS; Shah, HN; Finelli, FC; Carroll, NM; Kirkpatrick, JR; Koch, TR. Calcium deficiency is associated with small intestinal bacterial overgrowth after Roux-en-Y gastric bypass surgery. *Am J Gastroenterol* 2007; 102(S2): S202.
[37] Mechanick, JI; Youdim, A; Jones, DB; et al. Clinical practice guidelines for the perioperative nutritional, metabolic, and nonsurgical support of the bariatric surgery patients—2013 update: cosponsored by American Association of Clinical Endocrinologists, The Obesity Society, and American Society for Metabolic & Bariatric Surgery. *Obesity* 2013; 21: S1–S27.

[38] Bal, BS; Koch, TR; Finelli, FC; Sarr, MG. Management of medical and surgical disorders after divided Roux-en-Y gastric bypass surgery. *Nat Rev Gastroenterol Hepatol* 2010; 7(6): 320-334.

[39] Institute of Medicine (US) Standing Committee on the Scientific Evaluation of Dietary Reference Intakes. Dietary reference intakes for calcium, phosphorus, magnesium, vitamin D, and fluoride. Washington (DC): National Academies Press (US); 1997.

[40] Carolyn, ME; Vadim, S. Vitamin D supplementation efficacy: Sleeve gastrectomy versus gastric bypass surgery. *Obes Surg* 2014; 24(12): 2055-60.

[41] Dawson-Hughes, B; Heaney, RP; Holick, MF; Lips, P; Meunier, PJ; Vieth, R. Estimates of optimal vitamin D status. *Osteoporos Int* 2005; 16(7): 713-6.

[42] Al-Shoha, A; Qui, S; Palnitkar, S; et al. Osteomalacia with bone marrow fibrosis due to severe vitamin D deficiency after a gastrointestinal bypass operation for severe obesity. *Endocr Pract* 2009; 15(6): 528–33.

In: Bone Disorders, Screening and Treatment
Editor: Aubrey M. Stone
ISBN: 978-1-63482-155-1


Chapter 4

# Weight Status and Lean Body Mass Are Associated with Bone Mass and Bone Mineral Density among Adult Women

*Sylvia Kirchengast*[*]
University of Vienna, Department of Anthropology,
Vienna, Austria

## Abstract

Reduced bone mass, bone density and consequently the pathological conditions osteopenia and osteoporosis represent significant health problems and contribute to disability, mortality, and reduced health related quality of life among older women and men. Consequently the decline of bone mineral content (BMC) and bone mineral density (BMD) are mainly seen as aspects of ageing. Bone loss however may also occur among young people. An important risk factor is low weight status. Especially extreme slenderness in combination with malnutrition such among people suffering from eating disorders may accelerate bone turnover and may result in osteopenia and osteoporosis. The present study examines the impact of weight status – classified by Body mass index (BMI) categories defined by the WHO, but also of soft tissue body composition parameters such as body fat and muscle mass on bone mineral content and bone density among 864 Austrian women ageing between 20 and 88 years. Body composition as well as bone density is determined by dual energy x-ray absorptiometry (DXA). A marked impact of weight status and soft tissue body composition on bone density and bone mineral content could be observed for all age groups. This association of low weight status and low bone mass could be proved especially for young women suffering from eating disorders.

[*] Corresponding author: Prof. Dr. Sylvia Kirchengast, University of Vienna, Faculty of Life Sciences, Department of Anthropology, Althanstrasse 14, A-1090 Vienna, Austria. E-mail: sylvia.kirchengast@univie.ac.at.

**Keywords:** weight status, bone mass, bone mineral density, body composition

# Introduction

Osteoporosis is the most common human metabolic bone disease and is characterized by accelerated bone loss (Sambrook and Cooper 2006). Bone loss consequently results in increased bone fragility and enhances the risk of fatal fractures (Ensrud et al. 2007, Binkley 2009, Cawthon et al. 2009, Frisoli et al. 2011, Gielen et al. 2011). One in three women and one in five men is predicted to suffer from osteoporosis-related fractures in their lifetime (Keen 2007). Since fractures - first of all hip fractures - contribute to morbidity, disability, severely reduced health related quality of life and in the worst case mortality, osteoporosis impose not only a major medical problem but also an enormous social and economic burden for societies and states.

As a consequence various strategies for treatment but also for prevention of osteoporosis have been developed (WHO 1998). In order to prevent or treat pathologically reduced bone mass and bone density effectively its etiology must be understand. On cellular level, osteoporosis and bone loss are the results of an imbalance in the activity of osteoblasts and osteoclasts. In particular proliferation, differentiation and activity of osteoclasts are increased while osteoblast function is reduced and do not fully balance the effect of osteoclasts. As a consequence bone loss occurs (Sambrook and Cooper 2006). But which factors increase osteoclast activity and reduce osteoblast activity? Bone loss is mostly interpreted in line of the general ageing process. In particular reduced stem cell population produces fewer osteoblasts, calcium absorption is disturbed and the Vitamin D levels decrease (Keen 2007). On the other hand hormonal changes such as menopausal transition in women lead to reduced estrogen levels which enhance osteoclast activity and bone turnover.

Additionally bone loss may be promoted by a lack of physical activity, malnutrition, use of glucocorticoids but also nicotine and alcohol consumption (Sambrook and Cooper 2006). These life style associated risk factors may accelerate bone loss during young age, too. While the effects of the aging process and adverse lifestyle patterns on bone loss are widely accepted, the impact of weight status and soft tissue body composition on bone loss is still discussed controversial.

On the one hand body weight has been shown as a strong predictor of bone density and bone mass among children and adolescents (Bakker et al. 2003, El Hage et al. 2009, El Hage 2013) but also among elderly and postmenopausal women (Kirchengast et al. 2001a, Shapes et al. 2007, Gennaro et al. 2010, Skrzek et al. 2014). First of all a protective effect of overweight and obesity against osteoporosis was assumed, however this commonly held belief has been challenged by some authors (Kim et al. 2010).

Commonly accepted is the observation that extremely low weight status such as among patients suffering from Anorexia nervosa, is associated with dramatically decreased bone mass and bone density (Powers 1999, Hofman et al. 2009, Fazeli and Klibanski 2014).

On the other hand there is no consensus regarding the impact of soft tissue body composition such as fat mass, fat distribution, and lean body mass on bone mass and bone density (Traquini et al. 1997, Kirchengast et al. 2001b, Farr et al. 2010, Baker et al. 2013, Liu et al. 2011, Gomez –Cabello et al. 2013, Kirchengast and Huber 2012, 2013, Ilich et al. 2014,

Mosca et al. 2014). A strong positive relationship between lean body mass and bone mineral density was described by Gjesdal et al. (2008), Genaro et al. (2010) and Lima et al. (2009). Wang et al. (2005) reported a positive correlation between fat mass as well as lean body mass and bone mineral density (aBMD) at all skeletal sites but the effect of fat mass on BMD was noted to be smaller than that of lean body mass. While Tarquini et al. (1997) observed a major impact of fat distribution patterns on bone mass among postmenopausal women, Gomez-Cabello et al. (2013) interpreted the association between fat mass and bone mass among elderly women as mediated by the independent association between lean mass and bone mass.

Mosca et al. (2014) in contrast, reported a negative effect of body fat mass and body weight on bone mass among adolescents. The aim of the present study was to analyze the effect of weight status but also absolute and relative soft tissue body composition, in particular fat mass and lean body mass on bone density and bone mineral content among adult women.

# Subjects and Methods

## Study Design and Subjects

This study contains two sub-studies. Both were part of a larger project focusing on association patterns between soft tissue body composition and bone mass as well as bone mineral density (see acknowledgements). Sub-study 1 included 824 healthy women ranging in age from 20 to 88 years ($\bar{x}$=49.2 ± 12.8). About 1000 women were recruited by newspaper advertising and broadcasting, all of them were Austrians originating from Vienna or neighbouring Lower Austria. After extensive documentation of individual medical history, history of diseases, current and past medication and reproductive history, actual habitual physical activity was evaluated by means of the physical activity questionnaire by Baecke et al. (1982). Life time physical activity was assessed by an extended interview documenting life time history of regular physical activities from multiple sources including occupational physical activity and leisure time physical activity. Professional athletes were excluded from this analysis because the high level of physical activity is associated with improved muscle mass and bone density even during old age (Andreoli et al. 2012).

Further exclusion criteria were nicotine consumption, acute diseases or a history of chronic or metabolic bone disease, hip or knee replacements or suffering from physical disabilities. Furthermore persons who received cortisone medication or other hormonal therapy which might influence bone density and soft tissue body composition were excluded from investigation.

After this screening 824 women were included in the sample. This sample was divided into 5 age groups. Age group 1 comprised 96 healthy young adult women ageing between 20 and 30 years. Age group 2 comprised 254 healthy premenopausal women ageing between 30 and 49 years. 310 women were classified as postmenopausal group (age group 3) ageing between 50 and 59 years. Elderly women ageing 60 years and older were classified as "younger elderly" ageing between 60 and 75 years (n=116) and very old aged ageing 75 years and more (Age group 5 n=48). All elderly participants lived in private homes and not in residential care homes for the elderly.

None of them was dependent on homecare attendants or family members for normal activities of daily live. From a socioeconomic viewpoint the sample was homogeneous. All subjects belonged to the social middle class typical of urban Vienna.

Socioeconomic position was determined by means of a structured questionnaire including questions regarding marital status, educational level, profession or profession before retirement, family income and the geographical area of residence in Vienna. Sub-study 2 included 20 young women between the ages 19 and 25 years ($\bar{x}$=22.9 ± 2.8) suffering from Anorexia nervosa and 20 age matched healthy controls. The anorectic participants were selected according to the DSM IV criteria (APA 1994). All of them were of restricting type of Anorexia nervosa and suffered from secondary amenorrhoea. Binge eaters and purging types were excluded from the sample. 20 healthy female students of the University of Vienna with no history of eating disorders served as healthy controls.

Data collection took place at the Menox out-patient department for the treatment of climacteric symptoms in Vienna. All participants were informed about the objectives and methodology of the study and their right to withdraw at any time was explained. Strict confidentiality was ensured. The study was conducted in compliance with "Ethical principles for medical research involving human subjects" of the Helsinki Declaration.

## Somatometrics and Body Composition Analyses

Body height was measured to the nearest 0.5cm using a standard anthropometer and body weight to the nearest 0.1kg on a balance beam scale. Body mass index (BMI) kg/m$^2$ was calculated. Weight status classification was based on body mass index (BMI) kg/m$^2$ categories recommended by the WHO (1995):

BMI < 18.50: underweight
BMI 18.50- 24.99: normal weight
BMI 25.00-29.99: overweight
BMI 30.00-39.99: obese
BMI > 40.00 morbid obese

Body composition analysis was performed by dual-energy-x-ray absorptiometry (DXA) using a Hologic Delphi W scanner (Hologic Inc. Bedford, MA, US; software version 12.4.2).

Body composition was acquired from whole body scan following manufacturer for position, scan acquisition and analysis. The attenuation of x-rays dependent on the tissue composition, and absolute and relative fat mass and lean body mass are estimated. The scan time takes approximately 6 minutes and the radiation dose is low (0.1 mSievert). Default software readings provide lines positioned to divide separate body compartments such as head, upper and lower limbs and trunk. The lines were positioned always by the same trained person. According to Sakai et al. (2006) DXA (Delphi W) measures total bone mineral content (BMC) and bone mineral density (aBMD), total mass, absolute fat mass, relative fat mass (fat%) and lean soft tissue mass with a precision (coefficient of variation) of 0.1%, 1.5%, 1.1%, 0.5%, 1.1% and 0.8%, respectively.

All scans were obtained by the same person. Daily scanning of the manufacturer-supplied phantom confirmed no instrumentation drift.

Muscle mass was described by three different parameters: by the total lean body mass determined by DXA scans, but by additionally by appendicular skeletal muscle mass (ASM) to describe the muscle mass of the limbs. Appendicular skeletal muscle mass (ASM) was determined by combining the lean tissue mass of the regions of the arms and legs, excluding all other regions from analyses (Heymsfield et al. 1990). Since skeletal muscle mass is significantly related to stature height the relative ASM (RASM) was calculated as follows: ASM was divided by the square of height (metres squared).

Whole body bone density (aBMD total) and bone mass (BMC) were estimated by DXA measurements. In detail seven regional parameters of bone mineral content (BMC) were determined: total BMC, BMC of the head, BMC of the trunk, BMC of each arm, and BMC of each leg separately.

### Statistical Analyses

Statistical calculations were performed by using SPSS for Windows Program Version 18.0 (Microsoft corp.). After calculation of descriptive statistics (means, SDs) the Kolmogorov-Smirnov test was applied to test the somatometric and body composition variables for normal distribution. According to the results of the Kolmogorov Smirnov test a normal distribution could be assumed for all somatometric and body composition variables.

Partial correlations (age = constant) were calculated to analyse the relationship between aBMD as well as BMC and somatometric as well as body composition parameters.

To analyse the impact of weight status and soft tissue body composition on bone mineral content and bone density multiple regression analyses were performed.

Oneway Anova (Duncan test) and student t-tests were calculated to test group differences with respect to statistical significance. A probability P value of less than 0.05 was considered significant.

## Results

### Sub-Study 1

#### *Age Group Differences in Weight Status and Body Composition Parameters*

Weight status according to age group is presented in figure 1. With increasing age the amount of overweight and obesity increased significantly up to age group 4 (60 to 75 years). Thereafter the rate of overweight and obesity declined.

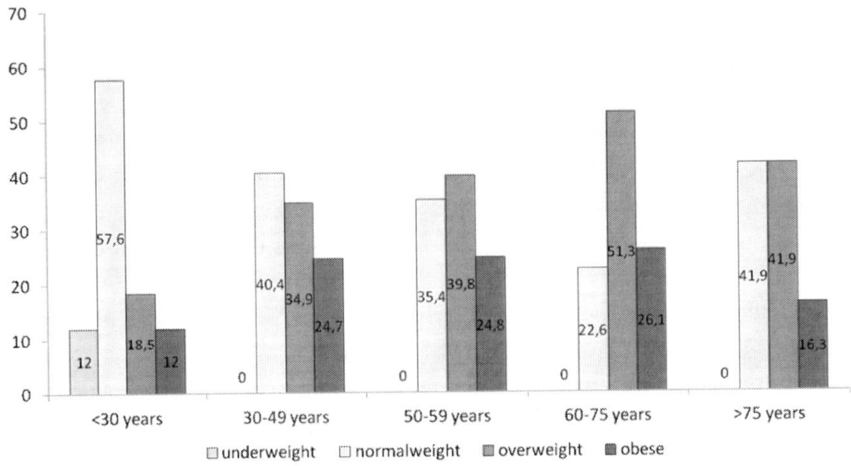


Figure 1. Weight status according to age group.

Table 1 presents age group differences in somatometric, soft tissue body composition, bone mineral content and bone density. While body height decreased significantly with increasing age, body weight and body mass index increased significantly up to age group 60 to 75 years. This steady increase up to age group 60 to 75 years was also true of absolute and relative fat mass. After 75 years bodyweight, weight status and absolute and relative fat mass declined. Lean soft tissue mass however started much earlier to decline.

Lean body mass of the whole body increased up to postmenopausal stage i.e. age group 50 to 60 years, absolute and relative appendicular muscle mass reached its peak between the ages of 30 and 49 years.

In contrast to soft tissue body composition and body weight, bone mineral content and bone density showed highest values among women younger than 30 years and decreased significantly with increasing age.

### *Weight Status and Bone Mass and Bone Density*

With increasing weight status bone mineral content increased significantly. This was true of all age groups. Bone mass of the whole body was always significantly lower among underweight or normalweight women in comparison to overweight or obese women (figure 2). Bone density was lowest among underweight and normal weight women and highest among obese women in all age groups with the exception of age group 1.

Among women younger than 30 years the bone density of obese women was significantly lower than that of overweight women (figure 3).

### *Predictors of aBMD and BMC*

Partial correlations (age = constant) of bone mineral content and bone density with somatometric and soft tissue body composition parameters are presented in table 2. Bone density (aBMD) correlated significantly positively with body height, body weight and all parameters of lean body mass.

**Table 1. Age group differences in somatometric parameters, body composition, bone density and weight status (ANOVA, Duncan test)**

| | < 30 years | 30-49 years | 50-60 years | 60-75 years | >75 years | |
|---|---|---|---|---|---|---|
| n | 96 | 254 | 310 | 116 | 48 | |
| | $\bar{x}$ (SD) | $\bar{x}$ (SD) | $\bar{x}$ (SD) | $\bar{x}$ (SD) | $\bar{x}$ (SD) | significance |
| Body height (cm) | 167.4 (5.9) | 165.5 (5.9) | 164.7 (5.6) | 163.2 (5.9) | 161.6 (4.9) | <0.001 |
| Body weight (kg) | 66.5 (16.3) | 73.4 (14.5) | 73.7 (12.6) | 74.4 (11.6) | 68.1 (11.6) | <0.001 |
| BMI (kg/m$^2$) | 23.72 (5.72) | 26.79 (5.21) | 27.19 (4.54) | 27.91 (3.85) | 26.11 (4.39) | <0.001 |
| Total Fat (kg) | 23.9 (13.0) | 31.4 (11.9) | 31.9 (9.2) | 33.7 (8.8) | 29.4 (9.5) | <0.001 |
| Fat (%) | 33.7 (10.1) | 40.7 (7.9) | 41.8 (7.2) | 43.6 (6.0) | 41.3 (7.2) | <0.001 |
| Total lean (kg) | 40.5 (4.9) | 41.1 (5.2) | 40.7 (4.4) | 40.1 (5.5) | 38.3 (3.9) | <0.001 |
| ASM (kg) | 16.5 (2.7) | 16.5 (2.7) | 16.1 (2.3) | 15.9 (2.6) | 15.0 (1.8) | <0.01 |
| RASM (kg/m$^2$) | 5.8 (0.9) | 6.0 (0.9) | 5.9 (0.8) | 5.9 (0.8) | 5.8 (0.7) | n.s. |
| BMC total (g) | 2308.4 (346.1) | 2304.7 (285.4) | 2270.2 (296.7) | 2107.9 (336.5) | 1868.9 (278.9) | <0.001 |
| BMC head (g) | 480.7 (77.6) | 478.7 (79.6) | 475.1 (90.1) | 432.5 (74.3) | 410.1 (65.4) | <0.001 |
| BMC right arm (g) | 155.7e (89.7) | 149.4e (25.2) | 148.9e (25.6) | 133.3e (30.1) | 114.3 (23.9) | <0.001 |
| BMC left arm (g) | 137.1 (32.3) | 134.9 (25.7) | 132.2 (28.7) | 117.5 (39.7) | 95.5 (27.9) | <0.001 |
| BMC trunk (g) | 645.4 (118.2) | 638.7 (106.2) | 623.7 (103.2) | 572.9 (131.6) | 507.4 (90.5) | <0.001 |
| BMC right leg (g) | 467.0 (71.8) | 456.3 (71.8) | 450.9 (66.1) | 430.5 (87.5) | 394.9 (83.9) | <0.001 |
| BMC left leg (g) | 457.6 (66.2) | 446.8 (78.2) | 444.4 (64.6) | 429.7 (92.6) | 382.2 (79.1) | <0.001 |
| aBMD total (g/m$^2$) | 1.11 (0.06) | 1.09 (0.09) | 1.09 (0.09) | 1.04 (0.11) | 1.00 (0.08) | <0.001 |

Legend: n.s. = not significant, ASM = appendicular skeletal mass, RASM = relative appendicular skeletal mass, BMI = body mass index, aBMD= bone mineral density, BMC = bone mineral content.

Absolute and relative body fat however showed no significant correlations with bone density. Concerning bone mineral content it turned out that body height, body weight, weight status but also absolute and relative fat mass as well as absolute and relative lean body mass correlated significantly positively with bone mass of all body compartments with the exception of the head.

To test the impact of age, weight status and soft tissue body composition parameters on bone density and bone mineral content of the whole body multiple regression analyses were performed. Multiple regression analyses indicated that age, weight status, and parameters of lean body mass were independently related to bone mineral density as well as to bone mineral content of the whole body. Absolute and relative fat mass however, had no significant impact on bone density and bone mineral content (table 3).

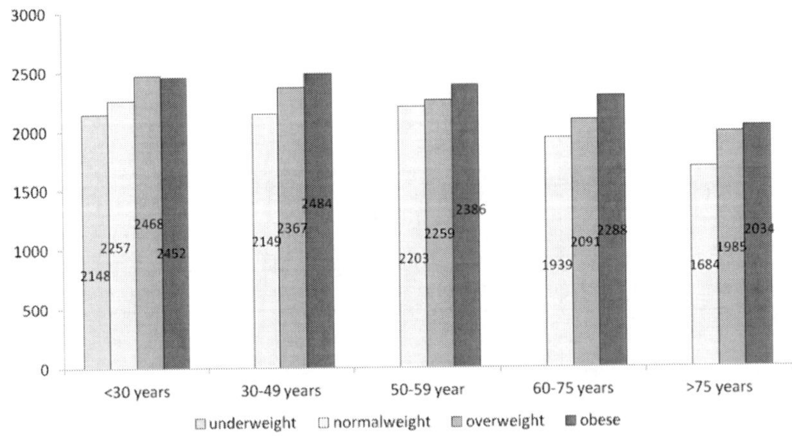


Figure 2. Total Bone mineral content (g) according to age group and weight status.

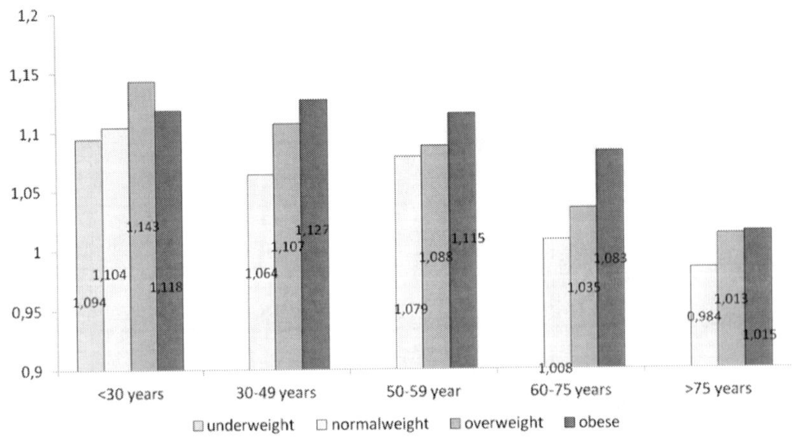


Figure 3. Areal Bone density (g/cm$^2$) according to age group and weight status.

## Sub-Study 2

To test the impact of low weight status and especially a low amount of body fat on bone, bone density and bone mineral content of twenty young women suffering from Anorexia nervosa were compared with those of healthy age matched controls.

**Table 2. Partial correlations (age=constant) of total bone mineral density (BMD), bone mass (BMC) and weight as well as body composition age**

| | Body height | Body weight | BMI | Total fat mass | Fat % | Total Lean body mass | ASM | RASM |
|---|---|---|---|---|---|---|---|---|
| aBMD total | 0.13** | 0.20*** | 0.15*** | 0.08 n.s. | -0.04 n.s. | 0.31*** | 0.28*** | 0.24*** |
| BMC total | 0.42*** | 0.48*** | 0.33*** | 0.34*** | 0.17*** | 0.56*** | 0.52*** | 0.36*** |
| BMC head | 0.17*** | -0.01 n.s. | -0.07 n.s. | -0.07 n.s. | -0.07 n.s. | 0.16** | 0.01 n.s. | 0.01 n.s. |
| BMC trunk | 0.39*** | 0.51*** | 0.37*** | 0.39*** | 0.22*** | 0.54*** | 0.49*** | 0.35*** |
| BMC right arm | 0.18*** | 0.24*** | 0.18*** | 0.17*** | 0.09* | 0.27*** | 0.25*** | 0.19*** |
| BMC left arm | 0.21*** | 0.26*** | 0.18*** | 0.14** | 0.17** | 0.36*** | 0.33*** | 0.26*** |
| BMC right leg | 0.47*** | 0.52*** | 0.34*** | 0.39*** | 0.23*** | 0.57*** | 0.55*** | 0.36*** |
| BMC left leg | 0.46*** | 0.49*** | 0.32*** | 0.37*** | 0.20*** | 0.53*** | 0.54*** | 0.35*** |

Legend: * $p < 0.05$; ** $p < 0.01$; *** $p < 0.001$. : n.s. = not significant, ASM = appendicular skeletal mass, RASM = relative appendicular skeletal mass, BMI = body mass index, aBMD= bone mineral density, BMC = bone mineral content.

Table 4 presents this comparison. As to be expected anorectic women showed significantly lower body weight, weight status, body fat mass and total lean body mass.

Absolute and relative appendicular muscle mass did not differ significantly between anorectic women and controls, although anorectic women showed always lower amounts of appendicular muscle mass. Furthermore no statistically significant differences in bone density, bone mineral content of the whole body and the legs could be observed. Bone mineral content of the trunk, including the spine and the arm however was significantly lower among anorectic women.

## Discussion

In the present study the impact of weight status and soft tissue body composition on bone mass and bone density among women ageing between 20 and 88 years was analyzed. Before starting to discuss the results in detail, it has to be stated that the present study has certain limitations.

**Table 3. Multiple regression models for predicting aBMD and BMC total**

| | Multiple R | Regression coefficient B | Significance | 95% confidence interval |
|---|---|---|---|---|
| Dependent variable: aBMD total | | | | |
| constant | 0.41 | 0.963 | <0.001 | 0.838 – 1.089 |
| Age | | -0.001 | 0.001 | -0.002 - -0.001 |
| BMI | | 0.010 | <0.01 | 0.004 -0.016 |
| Absolute fat mass | | -0.002 | n.s. | -0.005 – 0.001 |
| Fat% | | -0.002 | n.s. | -0.005 – 0.001 |
| Lean body mass | | 0.004 | <0.05 | - 0.007 |
| ASM | | 0.008 | n.s. | -0.003 – 0.020 |
| RASM | | -0.036 | <0.01 | -0.064 - -0.007 |
| Dependent variable: BMC total | | | | |
| Constant | 0.66 | 1177.992 | <0.001 | 828.169 -1527.816 |
| Age | | -4.957 | <0.001 | -6.295 - -3.619 |
| BMI | | 18.759 | <0.01 | 3.115 – 34.403 |
| Absolute Fat mass | | -1.188 | n.s. | -9.733 – 7.356 |
| Fat % | | 0.608 | n.s. | -7.214 -8.430 |
| Lean body mass | | 23.902 | <0.001 | 13.618 – 34.403 |
| ASM | | 81.343 | <0.001 | 49.289 – 113.396 |
| RASM | | 245.751 | <0.001 | 167.038 – 324.464 |

Legend: ASM = appendicular skeletal mass, RASM = relative appendicular skeletal mass, BMI = body mass index, aBMD= bone mineral density, BMC = bone mineral content.

One shortcoming is the small sample size (n=20) of sub-study 2 which results from the strict inclusion and exclusion criteria for anorectic participants. The other limitation is that bone mineral density was determined by DXA measurements and not by Computer tomography (CT). Therefore areal BMD and not volumetric BMD were determined. But nevertheless areal BMD is the most widely used densiometric parameter.

In a first step association patterns between weight status and bone mass as well as bone density were analysed. It could be shown that weight status, described by means of body mass index ($kg/m^2$) was significantly positively associated with bone mass as well as bone density. This was true of all age groups. This finding is in line with those of Chen et al. (1997), Kirchengast et al. (2002), Shapes et al. (2007) and Bredela et al. (2011).

Among the youngest age group (below 30 years) however, obese women showed a lower bone density and bone mass than overweight women. This observation is similar to that of Skrzek et al. (2014) who reported the lowest risk of bone loss for the interval 26.0 to 27.9 units of body mass index. This interval corresponds to the definition of overweight. The positive effect of higher weight status on bone mass and density was interpreted in two ways since the 1970s. On the one hand a protective effect of mechanical loading caused by weight bearing stress on bone density was postulated (Doyle et al. 1970). On the one hand hormonal factors as mediators were discussed. According to Shiraki et al. (1991) bone density in obese females is supported by higher serum levels in calcitonin, DHEA, DHEA-S, androstendione and testosterone.

**Table 4. Somatometric parameters, body composition, bone mass and bone density among young anorectic women and healthy controls (student t-test)**

| | Anorectic women | Healthy controls | |
|---|---|---|---|
| n | 20 | 20 | |
| | $\bar{x}$ (SD) | $\bar{x}$ (SD) | p-value |
| Body height (cm) | 168.2 (4.5) | 168.5 (5.7) | n.s. |
| Body weight (kg) | 48.9 (4.8) | 58.6 (9.1) | <0.001 |
| BMI (kg/m$^2$) | 17.34 (1.2) | 20.61 (2.37 | <0.01 |
| Total Fat (kg) | 10.2 (3.2 | 16.1 (4.8 | <0.001 |
| Fat (%) | 19.9 (5.5) | 27.1 (4.4) | <0.001 |
| Total lean (kg) | 36.7 (2.8) | 40.4 (4.8) | <0.05 |
| ASM (kg) | 15.4 (2.2) | 16.9 (3.1) | n.s. |
| RASM (kg/m$^2$) | 5.5 (0.7) | 5.9 (0.8) | n.s. |
| BMC total (g) | 2113.9 (233.1) | 2223.2 (245.2) | n.s. |
| BMC head (g) | 495.4 (77.6) | 461.4 (79.4) | n.s. |
| BMC right arm (g) | 118.3 (22.1) | 144.1 (23.8) | <0.01 |
| BMC left arm (g) | 115.1 (17.9) | 136.8 (19.3) | <0.01 |
| BMC trunk (g) | 555.7 (78.9) | 627.4 (91.1) | <0.05 |
| BMC right leg (g) | 417.6 (57.5) | 432.6 (67.5) | n.s. |
| BMC left leg (g) | 414.9 (57.3) | 420.9 (56.1) | n.s. |
| aBMD total (g/m$^2$) | 1.11 (0.07) | 0.98 (0.06) | n.s. |

Legend: n.s. = not significant, ASM = appendicular skeletal mass, RASM = relative appendicular skeletal mass, BMI = body mass index, aBMD= bone mineral density, BMC = bone mineral content.

More recently the strong association between adipose tissue and estrogen levels, which are a major determinant of trabecular microstructure among postmenopausal women, was interpreted as main reason of the positive effects of body weight on bone mass and bone density (Shapes et al. 2007). On the other hand excessive obesity enhances the secretion of inflammatory cytokines which may increase bone resorption and consequently bone loss (Smith et al. 2006). Contrary underweight has a clearly negative effect on bone mass and bone density, which could be demonstrated by analysing the anorectic subgroup. Anorectic young women showed a reduced bone mass and bone density in comparison to healthy normal weighted controls. This observation is in accordance with that of Powers (1999), Hofman et al. (2009) and Fazeli and Klibanski (2014). Severe underweight reduces biomechanical forces in the skeleton but also leads to reduced estrogen levels. Both may enhance bone loss.

Focusing on the impact of soft tissue body composition on bone mass and bone density we have to distinguish between lean mass or muscle mass and body fat. In the present study absolute and relative fat mass as well as absolute and relative lean body mass correlated highly significantly positively with bone mass and bone density independent of age. Considering the independent impact of body composition parameters on bone mass and bone density however, it could be shown that only lean body mass had an independent effect on bone mass and bone density. This observation is in line with the results of Gomez-Cabello et al. (2013) who reported that the association between fat mass and bone mass was mediated by the independent association between lean mass and bone mass. Fat mass -although an indicator of estrogen levels in women – seem to have only a minor positive impact on bone mass and bone density. Other studies revealed even a negative effect of fat mass on bone mass (Mosca et al. 2014).

In contrast to fat mass lean body mass or muscle mass had a significant positive impact on bone mass and bone density. This finding is in accordance with those of several previous studies (Kirchengast et al. 2001b, Lim et al. 2004, Lima et al. 2009, Gennaro et al. 2010, Kirchengast and Huber 2012, 2013, IT). According to Lang (2011) the skeletal muscle is one of the most powerful determinants of bone strength and bone density. A bone-muscle relationship was postulated and mainly viewed in the context of the mechanostat theory (Frost 1987, 2000) and the theory of the functional muscle bone unit (Schoenau 2005, Fricke and Schoenau 2007, Fricke et al. 2010). According to this theory bones respond to varying mechanical strains modulated by systemic effects such as hormones.

On the other hand bone and muscle have a common embryogenesis and both components are are regulated and controlled by the same hormones and genes (Matsuoka et al. 2005; Sayer and Cooper 2005; Karasik and Kiel 2010). Consequently the positive association between lean body mass and bone mass but also bone loss and muscle wasting are but two sides of the same coin because bone and muscle share genetic but also environmental, paracrine and endocrine influences throughout life (Karasik and Kiel 2010). The functional muscle bone unit was mainly described for children, adolescents and young adults (Schoenau 2005, Fricke and Schoenau 2007, Fricke et al. 2010, Ashby et al. 2011), while only few studies focused on the muscle-bone unit during adulthood and especially older age (Ferretti et al. 1998, 2003, Sumnik et al. 2006, Bleicher et al. 2011, Kirchengast and Huber 2012, 2013).

Nevertheless bone mass and skeletal muscle mass and are interrelated throughout life (Di Monaco et al. 2007, 2011; Walsh et al. 2006). According to the mechanostat theory muscle contractions induce tension in the bone, which in turn activates bone modeling via osteocyte mechanoreceptors (Frost 2003, Zofkova 2008). According the theory of a functionally unified muscle bone system, a healthy skeleton is adapted to mechanical stress as muscle tension leads to an increase in bone mass and strength (Fricke and Schoenau 2007).

Although bone loss and osteoporosis are mainly seen as a pathological condition of old age bone mass and bone density are effected by throughout life. Even during childhood and adolescence body weight but also soft tissue body composition parameters effect bone mass and bone density. During adolescence increasing levels of sex hormones enhance bone growth and peak bone mass and density is achieved at the end of third decade of life.

Stress factors such as extremely low body weight as in case of malnutrition, starvation or restrictive eating disorders reduced bone mass and bone density. Additionally typical life style parameters such as low physical activity levels, smoking or alcohol consumption but also medication such as cortisone treatment reduce bone growth during adolescence and early adulthood. Both, malnutrition and adverse life style parameters may result in a lower bone mass per se.

Starting with the fourth decade of life both sexes start to lose bone mass, a process which accelerates after menopause in women. The age related decline in bone mass and bone density is influenced by sex hormone levels (Greendale et al. 1997, Balasch 2003, Binkley 2009, Clarke and Khosla 2010, Gielen et al. 2011; Lang 2011), but also body composition parameters (Kirchengast and Huber 2013) and weight status (Skrzel et al. 2014).

Therefore we can conclude that weight status and lean body mass are associated with bone mass and bone mineral density and that low weight status and a low amount of skeletal muscle mass contribute to bone loss throughout adult life.

## Acknowledgments

The author is gratefully indebted to the Menox outpatient department for its kind cooperation. Special thanks go to the participants for the cooperation. The project was financially supported by the Hochschul-Jubiläumsfond (Project number: 1667/2006).

## References

American Psychiatric Association. 1994. *Diagnostic and statistical manual of mental disorders*. 4th ed. US.

Andreoli, A., Celi, M., Volpe, S. L., Sorge, R., Tarantino, U. 2012. Long-term effect of exercise on bone mineral density and body composition in postmenopausal ex-elite athletes: a retrospective study. *Eur. J. Clin. Nutr*. 66: 69-74.

Ashby, R. L., Adams, J. E., Roberts, S. A., Mughal, M. Z., Ward, K. A. 2011. The muscle-bone unit of peripheral and central skeletal sites in children and young adults. *Osteoporos. Int*. 22: 121-132.

Baecke, J. A. H., Burema, J., Frijters, J. E. R. 1982. A short questionnaire for the measurement of habitual physical activity in epidemiological studies. *Am. J. Clin. Nutr*. 36: 936-942.

Baker, J. F., Davis, M., Alexander, R., Zemel, B. S., Mostoufi-Moab, S., Shults, J., Sulik, M., Schiferl, D. J., Leonard, M. B. 2013. Associations between body composition and bone density and structure in men and women across the adult age spectrum. *Bone* 53: 34-41.

Bakker, I., Twisk, J. W. R., Van Mechelen, W. 2003. Fat-free body mass is the most important body composition determinant of 10-yr longitudinal development of lumbar bone in adult men and women. *J. Clin. Endocinol. Metab*. 88: 2607-2613.

Balasch, J. 2003. Sex steroids and bone, current perspectives. *Hum. Reprod. Update* 9: 207-222.

Binkley, N. 2009. A perspective on male osteoporosis. *Best Pract. Res. Clin. Rheumatol*. 23: 755-768.

Bleicher, K., Cumming, R. G., Naganathan, V., Travison, T. G., Sambrook, P. N., Blyth, F. M., Handelsman, D. J., Le Couteur, D. G., Waite, L. M., Creasey, H. M., Seibel, M. J. 2011. The role of fat and lean mass on bone loss in older men: Findings from the CHAMP study. *Bone* 49: 1299-1305.

Bredella, M. A., Torrani, M., Thomas, B. J., Brick, D. J., Gerweck, A. V., Harrington, L. M., Breggia, A., Rosen, C. J., Müller, K. K. 2011. Determinants of bone mineral density in obese premenopausal women. *Bone* 48: 748-754.

Cawthon, P. M., Ensrud, K. E., Laughlin, G. A. 2009. Sex hormones and frailty in older men, the osteoporotic fractures in men (MrOS) study. *J. Clin. Endocrinol. Metab*. 94: 3806-3815.

Chen, Z., Lohman, T. C., Stini, W. A., Ritenbaugh, C., Aickin, M. 1997. Fat or lean tissue mass: which one is the major determinant of bone mineral mass in healthy postmenopausal women? *J. Bone Mineral Res.* 12: 144-151.

Clarke, B. L., Khosla, S. 2010. Female reproductive system and bone. *Arch. Biochem. Biophysics* 503: 118-128.

Di Monaco, M., Vallero, F., Di Monaco, R., Tappero, R., Cavanna, A. 2007. Skeletal muscle mass, fat mass, and hip bone mineral density in elderly women with hip fracture. *J. Bone Mineral Metab.* 25: 237-242.

Di Monaco, M., Vallero, F., Di Monaco, R., Tappero, R. 2011. Prevalence of sarcopenia and its association with osteoporosis in 313 older women following a hip fracture. *Arch. Gerontol. Geriatrics* 52:71-74.

Doyle, F., Brown, J., Lachance, C. 1970. Relations between bone mass and muscle weight. *Lancet* 1 391-401.

El Hage, R., Jacob, C., Moussa, E., Groussard, C., Pineau, J. C., Benhamou, C. L., Jaffre, C. 2009. Influence of the weight status on bone mineral content and bone mineral density in a group of Lebanese adolescent girls. *Joint Bone Spine* 76: 680-684.

El Hage, R. 2013. Influence of the weight status on hip bone mineral density in young males. *Science and Sports* 28: 318-324.

Ensrud, K. E., Wing, S. K., Taylor, B. C., Fink, H. A., Stone, K. L., Cauley, J. A., Tracy, J. K., Hochberg, M. C., Rodondi, N., Cawthon, M. 2007. Frailty and risk of falls, fracture and mortality in older women, the study of osteoporotic fractures. *J. Gerontol. Ser. A Biol. Sci. Med. Sci.* 62: 74-751.

Farr, J. N., Chen, Z., Lisse, J. R., Lohman, T. G., Going, S. B. 2010. Relationship of total fat mass to weight-bearing bone volumetric density, geometry and strength in young girls. *Bone* 46: 977-984.

Fazeli, P. K., Klibanski, A. 2014. Anorexia nervosa and bone metabolism. *Bone* 66: 39-45.

Ferretti, J. L., Capozza, R. F., Cointry, G. R., Garcia, S. L., Plotkin, H., Alvarez Filgueira, M. L., Zanchetta, J. R. 1998. Gender related differences in the relationship between densiometric values of whole body bone mineral content and lean body mass in humans between 2 and 87 years. *Bone* 22: 683-690.

Ferretti, J. L., Cointry, G. R., Capozza, R. F., Frost, H. M. 2003. Bone mass, bone strength, muscle-bone interactions, osteopenias and osteoporoses. *Mech. Ageing Develop.* 124: 269-279.

Fricke, O., Schoenau, E. 2007. The functional muscle bone unit: probing the relevance of mechanical signals for bone development in children and adolescents. *Growth Hormone IGF Res.* 17: 1-9.

Fricke, O., Beccard, R., Semler, O., Schoenau, E. 2010. Analyses of muscular mass and function: the impact on bone mineral density and peak muscle mass. *Pediatr. Nephrol.* 25: 2393-2400.

Frisoli, A. Jr, Chaves, P. H., McNeill Ingham, S. J., Fried, L. P. 2011. Severe osteopenia and osteoporosis, sarcopenia and frailty status in community-dwelling older women: Results from the Women´s health and aging Study (WHAS) II. *Bone* 48: 952-957.

Frost, H. M. 1987. Bone mass and the mechanostat: a proposal. *Anatom. Rec.* 219: 1-9.

Frost, H. M. 2000. Muscle, bone and the Utah paradigm: a 1999 overview. *Med. Sci. Sports Exercise* 32: 911-917.

Frost, H. M. 2003. Bone´s mechanostat: a 2003 update. *Anat. Rec. A Discov. Mol. Cell Evol. Biol.* 275: 1081-1101.

Genaro, P. S., Pereira, G. A. P., Pinheiro, M. M., Szejnfeld, V. L., Martini, L. A. 2010. Influence of body composition on bone mass in postmenopausal osteoporotic women. *Arch. Gerontol. Geriat.* 51: 295-298.

Gielen, E., Vanderschueren, D., Callewaert, F., Boonen, S. 2011.Osteoporosis in men. *Best Pract. Res. Clin. Endocrinol. Metab.* 25: 321-335.

Gjesdal, C. G., Halse, J. I., Eide, G. E., Brun, J. G., Tell, G. S. 2008. Impact of lean mass and fat mass on bone mineral density, The Hordaland Health Study. *Maturitas* 59: 191-200.

Gomez-Cabello, A., Ara, I., Gonzalez-Agüero, A., Casajus, J. A., Vicente-Rodriguiz, G. 2013. Fat mass influence on bone mass is mediated by independent association between lean mass and bone mass among elderly women: Across-sectional study. *Maturitas* 74: 44-53.

Greendale, G. A., Edelstein, S., Barrett-Connor, E. 1997. Endogeneous sex steroids and bone mineral density in older women and men. The Rancho Bernardo Study. *J. Bone Mineral Res.* 12: 1833-1843.

Heymsfield, S. B., Smith, R., Aulet, M., Bensen, B., Lichtman, S., Wang, J., Pierson, R. N. 1990. Appendicular skeletal muscle mass, measurements by dual-photon absorptiometry. *Am. J. Clin. Nutr.* 52: 214-218.

Hofman, M., Landewe-Cleuren, S., Wojciechowski, F., Nieuwenhuijzen Kruseman, A. 2009. Prevalence and clinical determinants of low bone mineral density in anorexia nervosa. *Europ. J. Internal Med.* 30: 88-84.

Ilich, J. Z., Kelly, O. J., Inglis, J. E., Panton, L. B., Duque, G., Ormsbee, M. J. 2014. Interrelationship among muscle, fat and bone: Connecting the dots on cellular, hormonal and whole body levels. *Ageing Res. Rev.* 15: 51-60.L

Karasik, D., Kiel, D. P. 2010. Evidence for pleiotropic factors in genetics of musculoskeletal system. *Bone* 46: 1226-1237.

Keen, R. 2007. Osteoporosis: strategies for prevention and management. *Best Practice and Res. Clin. Rheumatol.* 21: 109-122.

Kim, K. C., Shin, D. H., Lee, S. Y. Im, J. A., Lee, D. E. 2010. Relation between obesity and bone mineral density and vertebral fractures in Korean postmenopausal women. *Yosei Med. J.* 51: 857-863.

Kirchengast, S., Peterson, B., Hauser, G., Knogler, W. 2001a. Zur Bedeutung des Gewichtsstatus für die Knochendichte bei Betagten und Hochbetagten. *Zeitschr. Gerontol.* 34: 1-6.

Kirchengast, S., Peterson, B., Hauser, G., Knogler, W. 2001b. Body composition characteristics are associated with the bone density of the proximal femur end in middle- and old aged women and men. *Maturitas* 39: 133-145.

Kirchengast, S., Knogler, W., Hauser, G. 2002. Protective effect of moderate overweight on bone density of the hip joint in elderly and old Austrians. *Anthrop. Anz.* 60: 187-197.

Kirchengast, S., Huber, J. 2012. Sex specific associations between soft tissue body composition and bone mineral density among older adults. *Ann. Hum. Biol.* 39: 206.

Kirchengast, S., Huber, J. 2013. Age typical associations between skeletal muscle mass and bone mass among healthy women. *J. Women's Health Issues and Care 2.*

Lang, T. F. 2011. The bone muscle relationship in men and women. *J. Osteoporos.* doi:10.4061/2011/702735.

Lim, S., Joung, H., Dhin, C. S., Lee, H. K., Kim, K. S., Shin, E. K., Kim, H. Y., Lim, M. K., Cho, S. I. 2004. Body composition changes with age have gender specific impacts on bone mineral density. *Bone* 35: 792-798.

Lima, R. M., Bezerra, L. M. A., Rabelo, H. T., Silva, M. A. F., Silva, A. J. R., Bottaro, M., de Oliviera, R. J. 2009. Fat-free mass, strength and sarcopenia are related to bone mineral density in older women. *J. Clin. Densiometry* 12: 35-41.

Liu, S., Li, J., Sheng, Z., Wu, X., Liao. 2011. Relationship between body composition and age, menopause and its effects on bone mineral density at segmental regions in Central Southern Chinese postmenopausal elderly women with and without osteoporosis. *Arch. Gerontol. Geriatrics* 53: e192-3197.

Matsuoka, T., Ahlberg, P. E., Kessaris, N., Iannrelli, P., Dennehy, U., Richardson, W. D., McMahon, A. P., Koentges, G. 2005. Neural crest origins of the neck and shoulder. *Nature* 436: 347-355.

Mosca, L., Lederer Goldberg, T. B., da Silva, V. N., da Silva, C. C., Kurokawa, C. S., Rizzo, A. C. B., Corrente, J. E. 2014. Excess body fat negatively effects bone mass in adolescents. *Nutrition* 30: 847-852.

Powers, P. S. 1999. Osteoporosis and eating disorders. *J. Pediatr. Adolesc. Gynecol.* 12: 51-57.

Sakai, Y., Ito, H., Meno, T., Numata, M., Jingu, S. 2006. Comparison of body composition measurements obtained by two fan-beam DXA instruments. *J. Clin. Densiometry* 9: 191-197.

Sambrook, P., Cooper, C. 2006. Osteoporosis. *The Lancet* 367: 2010-2018.

Sayer, A. A., Cooper, C. 2005. Fetal programming of body composition and musculoskeletal development. *Early Human Develop.* 81: 735-744.

Schoenau, E. 2005. From mechanostat theory to development o of the functional muscle bone unit. *J. Musculoskelet. Neuronal Interact.* 5: 232-238.

Schoenau, E., Neu, C. M., Beck, B., Manz, F., Rauch, F. 2002. Bone mineral content per muscle cross-sectional area as an index of the functional muscle-bone unit. *J. Bone Mineral Res.* 17: 1095-1101.

Shapes, S. A., Riedt, C. S., Schlussel, Y., Gordon, C. L., Li, W. P., Brolin, R. E., Stahl, T. 2007. Body weight and menopausal status influence trabecular and cortical bone mineral density. *Int. Congress Series* 1297: 231-240.

Shiraki, M., Ito, H., Fujimaki, H., Higucji, T. 1991. Relation between body size, and bone mineral density with special reference to sex hormones and calcium regulating hormones in elderly females. *Endocrinol. Jap.* 38: 343-349.

Skrzek, A., Koziel, S., Ignasiak, Z. 2014. The optimal value of BMI for the lowest risk of osteoporosis in postmenopausal women aged 40 – 88 years. *Homo* 65: 232-239.

Smith, B. J., Lerner, M. R., Bu, S. Y., Lucas, E. A., Hanas, J. S., Lightfoot, S. A., Postier, R. G., Bronze, M. S., Brackett, D. J. 2006. Systematic bone loss and induction of coronary vessel disease in a rat model of chronic inflammation. *Bone* 38: 378-386.

Sumnik, Z., Land, C., Coburger, S., Neu, C., Manz, F., Hrach, K., Schoenau, E. 2006. The muscle bone unit in adulthood: influence of sex, height, age and gynecological history on the bone mineral content and muscle cross sectional area. *J. Muskuloskelet. Neuronal Interact.* 6: 195-200.

Tarquini, B., Navari, N., Perfetto, F., Piluso, A., Romano, S., Tarquini, R. 1997. Evidence for bone mass and body fat distribution relationhip in postmenopausal obese women. *Arch. Gerontol. Gereatrics* 24: 15-21.

Walsh, M. C., Hunter, G. R., Livingstone, M. B. 2006. Sarcopenia in premenopausal and postmenopausal women with osteopenia, osteoporosis and normal bone mineral density. *Osteoporosis Int.* 17: 61-67.

Wang, M. C., Bachrach, L. K., Van Loan, M., Hudes, M., Flegal, K. M., Crawford, P. B. 2005. The relative contributions of lean tissue mass and fat mass to bone density in young women. *Bone* 37: 474-481.

WHO 1995. Physical status: the use and interpretation of anthropometry. *WHO Techn. Rep. Ser. 854. Genf.*

WHO. 1998. Assessment of fracture risk and its application to screening for postmeopausal osteoporosis. *Technical Report Series 843*. Geneva.

Zofkova, I. 2008. Hormonal aspects of the muscle bone unit. *Physiol. Res.* 57: S159-S169.

In: Bone Disorders, Screening and Treatment
Editor: Aubrey M. Stone

ISBN: 978-1-63482-155-1


*Chapter 5*

# Alcohol and Bone Health: A Review

***J. J. Zhang[1], M. Clynes[1], G. Robinson[2], C. Cooper[1,3] and E. M. Dennison*[1,4]***

[1]MRC Lifecourse Epidemiology Unit, University of Southampton, UK
[2]Capital and Coast District Health Board Wellington, New Zealand
[3]NIHR Musculoskeletal Biomedical Research Unit,Nuffield Department of Orthopaedics, Rheumatology and Musculoskeletal Science, University of Oxford, UK
[4]Victoria University, Wellington, New Zealand

## Abstract

Regular alcohol consumption is now widespread with public health concerns regarding the effect of excessive intake on all groups. This review considers the relationship between different levels of alcohol intake and bone health among adolescent, pre and post-menopausal women and men, and will discuss the possible mechanisms of alcohol's influence on bone health. In general, regular low levels of alcohol consumption are associated with above average bone mineral density (BMD), while excessive alcohol consumption is associated with reduced BMD possibly through a direct toxic effect on bone turnover but also through associated lifestyle factors.

## Introduction

Since the early studies performed by Laitinen and Valimaki in 1991 [1] highlighting both the deleterious and beneficial effects of alcohol on bone, there has been a wealth of research considering this topic. The importance of the effect of lifestyle factors on bone health is of

* Correspondence and reprint requests to: Prof Elaine Dennison, MRC Lifecourse Epidemiology Unit, Southampton General Hospital, Southampton, SO16 6YD, UK; Telephone: 023 8077 7624, Fax: 023 8070 4021, Email: emd@mrc.soton.ac.uk.

major public health importance, given the burden of osteoporosis and its consequences [2]. Currently it is estimated that more than 75 million people in Europe, Japan and the USA are affected by osteoporosis, and annually more than 2.3 million fractures in Europe and the USA are osteoporosis related [3]. This review will explore the possible mechanisms involved in the effect of alcohol on bone, and review the epidemiological evidence of an effect of alcohol on the bone mass of men, premenopausal and post-menopausal women, and adolescents.

## Interaction between Alcohol and Bone Health (Aetiopathogenesis)

The effect alcohol has on the health of bones is multifactorial.

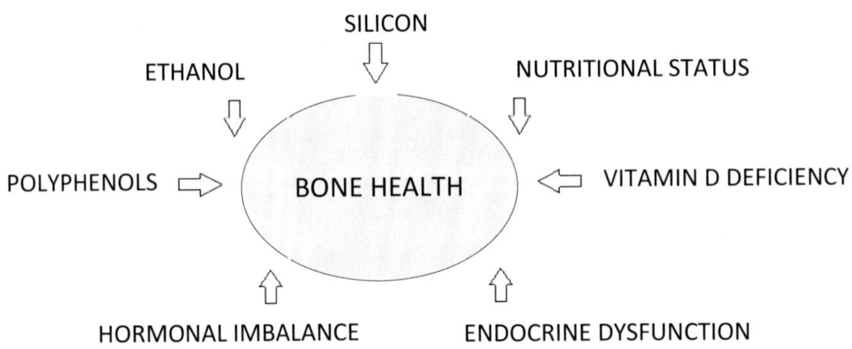


## Direct Effect of Ethanol, Silicon and Polyphenols

Alcoholic beverages typically contain a mixture of ethanol, silicon and polyphenols, all of which have been shown to have an effect upon bone health. Ethanol has been shown in some cell culture studies to directly inhibit bone formation through an effect upon osteoblasts [4], although some studies have failed to demonstrate such an effect on matured osteoblasts [5]. Studies have often demonstrated a dose-dependent toxic effect [6].

By contrast dietary silicon (Si) has been shown to be positively associated with bone mineral density (BMD) in men and premenopausal women, particularly cortical bone [7]. Typically beer contains an average (mean) of 19.2mg/L (SD 6.6) of Si [8]while concentrations in wine are lower (fortified port wine having the lowest amount, 0.62mg/portion to rose wine with 2.89mg/portion) [9]. Si in alcoholic drinks such as beer is well absorbed with an absorption rate of approximately 55%, and quickly filtered by the kidneys, with an ultrafilterability of 80% [8].

Finally, phenolic compounds are also found in alcoholic drinks, particularly red wine, but also beer. It is possible that numerous potential signalling pathways regulating osteoblasts and osteoclasts may be impacted by these compounds; for example EGCG and resveratrol bind to the oestrogen receptors (α and β) exerting an oestrogenic effect [10]. Others have been found to regulate pathways that lead to activation of transcription factors such as NK-κB resulting in changes in proliferation, differentiation, and collagen formation [10].

High levels of alcohol intake appear negatively related to bone formation markers such as osteocalcin and tartrate-resistant acid phosphatase isoenzyme 5b [11]. This suppression appears to be reversible; a cohort of alcoholic male patients enrolled in a programme for abstinence for 8 weeks, showed a significant increase in osteocalcin (bone formation marker) levels from a lowered baseline level in 17% of the cohort, with concurrent observed elevated levels of crosslaps (a marker of bone resorption) in 34% of the cohort at baseline [12]. Likewise a study of 34 alcohol dependent of women mean age 41.7 (8.04) years admitted to an alcohol withdrawal unit observed that the marker of bone formation P1NP rose significantly over the detoxification programme [day 1: 28.35 μg/l (12.25); day 5: 34.19 μg/l (13.16), $p=0.003$] but CTX change was not significant [13].

## Nutritional Status and Vitamin D Deficiency

Alcoholic dependent individuals are vulnerable to nutritional deficits since the majority of the daily calorific intake is often taken up by alcohol [14]. Impaired nutritional status, and being undernourished (a lower lean body mass, and risk of magnesium and vitamin D deficiencies) [14, 15] are common observations in alcoholics [16]. Further insults can be added when these high risk patients develop liver pathologies and involvement of their gastrointestinal system resulting in malabsorption. Alcoholics are high risk in developing chronic pancreatitis which also contributes to the phenomenon of malabsorption syndrome. Vitamin D deficiency is common [15]; in a recent study researchers observed a much lower Vitamin D level 26.5 (IQR = 17.0-37.8 pg/ml) in heavy drinkers (>150g ethanol/day (204 ± 82 g/day)) compared to the control group of 82.4 (IQR = 60.9-107.4 pg/ml, $P < 0.001$) [6]. It has often been hypothesised that other lifestyle factors may confound the relationship between alcohol and bone where those who drink moderately may lead an otherwise healthier lifestyle [17, 18].

## Hormonal Effect and Endocrine/ Metabolic Disorder

Consumption of alcohol has been linked to increased conversion of androstenedione to oestrone and may also increase adrenal stimulation which has a positive effect on BMD [19]. Certainly this oestrogenic effect is seen in several studies [20-22], where the positive effect is seen in either men or post-menopausal women but not pre-menopausal women. Laitinen and Valimaki [1] highlighted the consequence of low vitamin D level which can lead to potentially poor absorption of calcium, which in turn can trigger high levels of circulating PTH. Raised levels of PTH is commonly observed in alcoholics [1], leading to further bone turnover and bone loss [23]. Alcohol induced Cushing's syndrome was initially mentioned in a series of case reports linking alcohol abuse with the symptoms and signs of Cushingoid patients [24].The effect of excessive cortisol is well known to affect bone health deleteriously. Finally male hypogonadism has often been reported as a consequence of alcohol excess [25], and in females secondary amenorrhoea with low level of oestradiol can occur [26].

## Men and Alcohol

Excessive drinking in men and the harmful effect on bone has been well established in epidemiological studies; however the effect of everyday consumption is less clear cut. Holbrook and Barrett-Connor [27] recruited 182 men to a study in which their 1 week of alcohol intake were recorded with thresholds defined as a mean of 46.2 (24.7-SD)g for low intake, 136.3 (26.9-SD)g for medium intake, 324.3 (115.5-SD)g for high intake; and BMD recorded at several sites. They found a statistically significant positive relationship between BMD and alcohol intake at the femoral neck and this relationship was also seen at all other sites but was not statistically significant. Additionally the increase in BMD associated with increased alcohol intake was independent of baseline age, BMI, smoking and regular exercise. Similar relationships were observed in the Framingham Study [20], where subjects consuming >14oz (414ml)/week had higher BMD at every site than non-drinkers, although this relationship did not reach statistical significance. In a nationally representative sample of the USA [28] after adjustment for other lifestyle factors, men who drank regular alcohol had 2% higher BMD at total hip and femoral neck sites than abstainers.

A recent meta-analysis reported on this topic (Figure 1) and observed a linear relationship between femoral neck and vertebral spine bone density and alcohol [29], although this included only 4 cohort papers. The relationship between bone loss over time and alcohol was also explored. Of the three studies included, two supported a U shaped relationship suggesting that regular modest consumption of alcohol (0.7-1.4/1.7 drinks per day) has the lowest bone loss over time compared with non-drinkers and those drinking more than 1.7 drinks per day. The final study observed no linear relationship between alcohol consumption and bone loss.

Studies carried out in recent years have yielded conflicting results. However several studies [11, 22, 30, 31] have indicated that consuming some alcohol is associated with a higher bone mass. By contrast a study of a cohort of elderly Australian men [32] that reported BMD at the forearm demonstrated an inverse relationship between bone health and alcohol intake.

Recent work by Paccou et al., (unpublished) employing high resolution computed tomography (HRPQCT) as a novel way of measuring bone health, found that men with a low (≥1 to <11 units/week) or moderate/high (≥11 units/week) alcohol consumption had lower cortical thickness, cortical density, trabecular thickness and trabecular BMD, than men who drank none/minimal (<1 unit/week) alcohol (Figure 2).

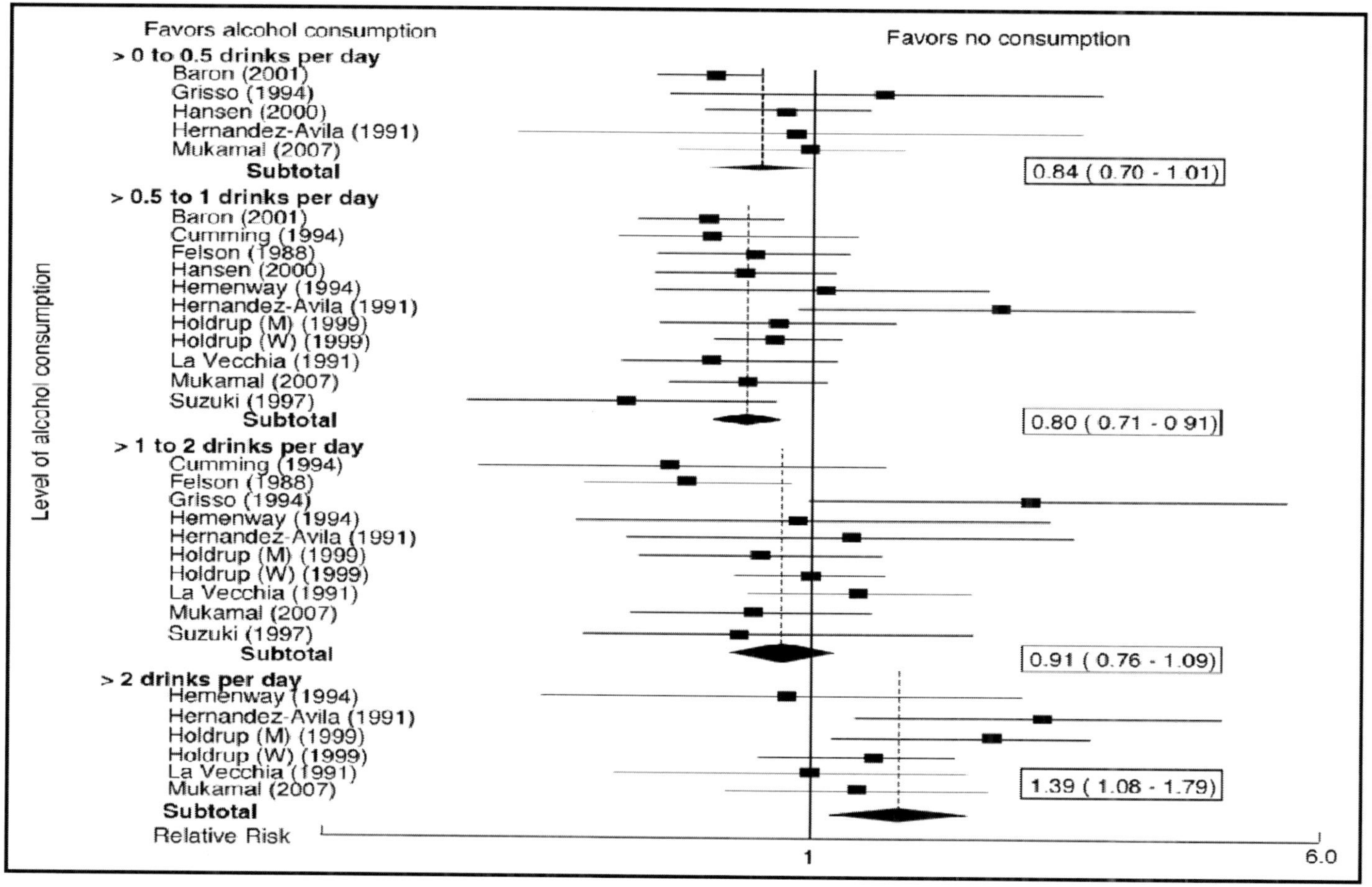


Figure 1. Association between alcohol consumption and hip fracture risk. Reference exposure is zero drinks per day. Size of data marker represents sample size. Horizontal lines denote 95% confidence intervals. (Reproduced with permission from reference 29).

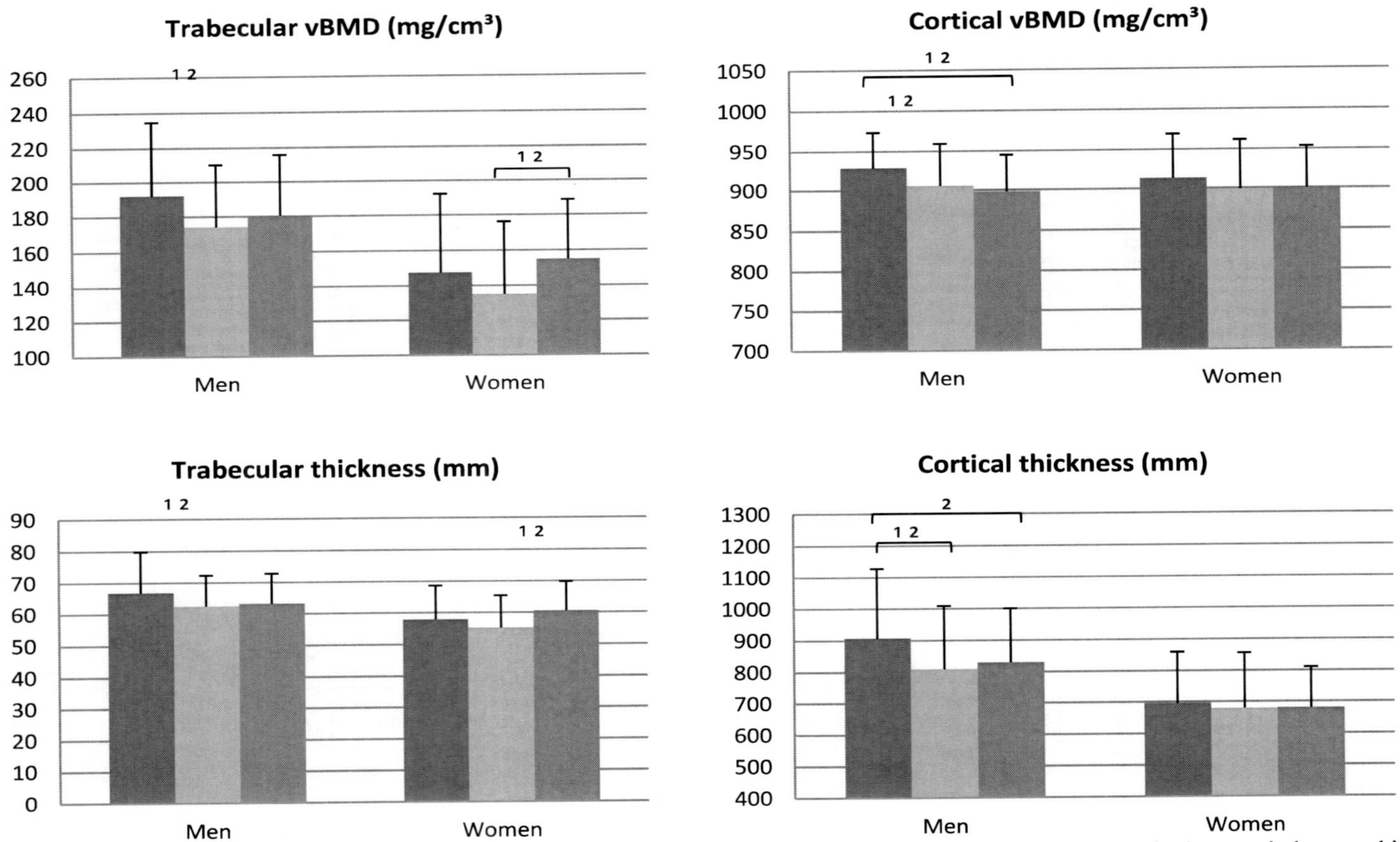


[1] indicate significant differences between alcohol consumption categories without adjustment and [2] with adjustment by age, body mass index, smoking status, calcium intake, physical activity and social class.

Figure 2. Comparative analysis of bone geometry, vBMD and microarchitecture in men and women on alcohol consumption.

Other studies have shown a similar thresholding effect. In a Japanese study, the threshold level of alcohol consumption positively associated with BMD was 55g/day [11] and beyond this level alcohol consumption was negatively associated with BMD. In the Framingham Osteoporosis Study [22], the optimal total alcohol intake was 1-2 drinks/day with this group having the highest BMD and beyond 2 drinks/day there was again a trend for lower BMD. More than 14 oz (414ml)/week was the figure suggested as a threshold in an earlier Framingham Study [20], and 12-21 units/week was the finding from a cohort of young UK Army recruits [33]. The variation in the units and numbers from all these studies make it difficult to precisely identify what is the optimal amount of alcohol with regards to BMD.

There have being some studies looking into the effects of alcohol on bone health in adolescents and young men. An inverse relationship between alcohol consumed (g/day) and BMD was seen in a group of young men aged 20-23 [34]. Similar relationships were observed in another cohort of students [35] where researchers found that any self-reported alcohol intake was associated with a lower BMD. Conversely, a cohort study of young UK Army recruits [33] found those with a moderate intake of alcohol (12-21 units/week) had higher BMDs, but once again, the highest consumption group (>21 units/week) has the lowest BMD, highlighting the deleterious effect alcohol can have when consumed in high amounts. Similarly, a large study of Norwegian adolescents [36], of mean age 16.82 (1.04-SD) years reported that boys who drank alcohol had higher BMD at all sites when compared with their teetotal peers.

## Premenopausal Women and Alcohol

In the Wisconsin study discussed previously, a lower BMD was also observed in the female half of the cohort with self-reported alcohol use [35]. Likewise in the largest study of alcohol consumption and bone health that includes adolescents to date, the researchers found a negative relationship between alcohol consumption overall on BMD [37]. This cohort study included 892 girls who were studied at the age of 17. In the same year [38] 262 girls aged 11-19 years, were studied and no association between alcohol and bone measures were found. It is possible the low usage of alcohol of the sample group may be a major contributor towards the lack of statistical findings.

By contrast, the large Norwegian adolescent study discussed above suggested that drinking alcohol was negatively associated with BMD in young women, although this trend did not reach statistical significances [36] suggesting that sexual dimorphism in the relationship between alcohol and bone may act in the teenage years.

Laitinen et al., [21] also studied the effect of alcohol on pre-menopausal women's BMD. Among 186 pre-menopausal Finnish women, no association was found between alcohol intake and BMD overall. Similarly in a study by Wosjie et al., [28] there were no statistically significant differences in BMD according to alcohol consumption.

Jugdaohsigh [10] highlighted the lack of consensus in the studies performed in premenopausal women, with some supporting the beneficial effect of moderate consumption of alcohol, whilst others finding the opposite and one study finding no effect at all.

Much of the epidemiological data relates to low levels of alcohol consumption in cohort studies. High levels of alcohol consumption in young women has been highlighted as a major public health concern, and is likely to lead to adverse effects of bone, although research is scanty in this area. In a recent case control study of women admitted to an alcohol withdrawal unit and healthy controls, of mean age 41.7 (8.04) years and 42.3 (12.95) years respectively, alcoholic women had lower heel ultrasound T scores [mean -1.2 (1.3)] compared with controls [mean -0.3 (1.4)] ($p=0.05$), but differences in other heel ultrasound results (BUA; SOS; SI) were of borderline significance. The marker of bone formation P1NP rose significantly over the detoxification programme [day 1: 28.35 µg/l (12.25); day 5: 34.19 µg/l (13.16), $p=0.003$] but CTX change was not significant. Of the alcoholic women who had circulating vitamin D results available, six (37.5%) had a circulating vitamin D level falling below the lower limit of normal (50nmol/l). Lifestyle factors associated with poor bone health, were prevalent in female alcoholics [13].

## Postmenopausal Women and Alcohol

Laitinen et al., [21] first reported a positive correlation between alcohol use and BMD in a modest sized group of 71 post-menopausal women, with a mean age of 59.1±6.4 years. Similar results have been replicated in different populations. A study of 2000 Chinese women aged ≥65 year old reported that alcohol consumption was positively associated with BMD at the hip and spine, despite having a relatively low number of drinkers in the cohort [39].

A Finnish study group, OSTPRE-FP [40], and the Aberdeen Prospective Osteoporosis Screening Study (APOSS) [41] both reported that BMD was greater in those who drank alcohol than non-drinkers; women consuming 3 drinks/week had 12% higher BMD at the femoral neck and 9.2% at lumbar spine than abstainers [40]. In the Framingham Study [20], women consuming ≥7oz alcohol /week had higher BMDs than those drinking <1oz/week. Similarly Tucker et al., [22] observed a threshold of >2 drinks/day for a beneficial effect on bone health. Of note this level of alcohol consumption is higher than what is considered to be moderate in the US. In addition, the overall positive trend seen in Tucker et al., [22] in all groups of drinkers, is stronger than the positive trend found in their male counterparts. Not all studies have found this positive correlation; Yin et al., [31] found that baseline BMD did not correlate with total alcohol intake (grams or drinks/day).

It has been suggested that the explanation for the positive relationship between modest alcohol consumption and bone health seen in post-menopausal women is confounded by other lifestyle factors, such as physical activity.

The Aberdeen Prospective Osteoporosis Screening Study (APOSS) [41] investigated this, and were unable to remove the positive associations they observed by adjustment for known lifestyle factors, but the possibility of residual confounding remains.

## Conclusion

It remains unclear what exact level of alcohol consumption is associated with an optimal effect on bone health. In general, the literature reports that modest alcohol consumption is associated with higher than average BMD, although it is unclear whether residual confounding is the explanation for this. High levels of alcohol consumption, above recommended levels, have been reported in several studies to be negatively associated with bone health, through a direct effect of alcohol and other compounds found in alcoholic beverages on bone mineral health, but also through associated lifestyle factors such as poor nutrition and cigarette smoking, and an increased rate of falls. Further research in this area is now required.

# References


[1] Laitinen K, Valimaki M. Alcohol and bone. Calcified tissue international. 1991;49 Suppl:S70-3. *PubMed PMID:* 1933604. Epub 1991/01/01. eng.

[2] Bone Health and Osteoporosis: A Report of the Surgeon General. Rockville MD2004.

[3] World Health Organisation. Prevention and Management of Osteoporosis: report of a WHO scientific group. Geneva, Switzerland2000.

[4] Turner RT. Skeletal response to alcohol. Alcoholism, clinical and experimental research. 2000 Nov;24(11):1693-701. PubMed PMID: 11104117. Epub 2000/12/05. eng.

[5] Klein RF, Carlos AS. Inhibition of osteoblastic cell proliferation and ornithine decarboxylase activity by ethanol. *Endocrinology.* 1995;136(8):3406-11. PubMed PMID: 7628376.

[6] Alvisa-Negrin J, Gonzalez-Reimers E, Santolaria-Fernandez F, Garcia-Valdecasas-Campelo E, Valls MR, Pelazas-Gonzalez R, et al. Osteopenia in alcoholics: effect of alcohol abstinence. Alcohol and alcoholism (Oxford, Oxfordshire). 2009 Sep-Oct;44(5):468-75. PubMed PMID: 19535494. Epub 2009/06/19. eng.

[7] Jugdaohsingh R, Tucker KL, Qiao N, Cupples LA, Kiel DP, Powell JJ. Dietary silicon intake is positively associated with bone mineral density in men and premenopausal women of the Framingham Offspring cohort. *Journal of bone and mineral research: the official journal of the American Society for Bone and Mineral Research.* 2004 Feb;19(2):297-307. PubMed PMID: 14969400. Epub 2004/02/19. eng.

[8] Sripanyakorn S, Jugdaohsingh R, Elliott H, Walker C, Mehta P, Shoukru S, et al. The silicon content of beer and its bioavailability in healthy volunteers. *The British journal of nutrition.* 2004 Mar;91(3):403-9. PubMed PMID: 15005826. Epub 2004/03/10. eng.

[9] Powell JJ, McNaughton SA, Jugdaohsingh R, Anderson SH, Dear J, Khot F, et al. A provisional database for the silicon content of foods in the United Kingdom. *The British journal of nutrition.* 2005 Nov;94(5):804-12. PubMed PMID: 16277785. Epub 2005/11/10. eng.

[10] Jugdaohsingh R, O'Connell MA, Sripanyakorn S, Powell JJ. Moderate alcohol consumption and increased bone mineral density: potential ethanol and non-ethanol mechanisms. *The Proceedings of the Nutrition Society.* 2006 Aug;65(3):291-310. PubMed PMID: 16923313. Epub 2006/08/23. eng.

[11] Kouda K, Iki M, Fujita Y, Tamaki J, Yura A, Kadowaki E, et al. Alcohol intake and bone status in elderly Japanese men: baseline data from the Fujiwara-kyo osteoporosis risk in men (FORMEN) study. *Bone.* 2011 Aug;49(2):275-80. PubMed PMID: 21530699. Epub 2011/05/03. eng.

[12] Malik P, Gasser RW, Moncayo R, Kemmler G, Wolfgang Fleischhacker W. Markers of bone resorption and formation during abstinence in male alcoholic patients. *Alcoholism, clinical and experimental research.* 2012 Dec;36(12):2059-64. PubMed PMID: 22978478. Epub 2012/09/18. eng.

[13] Dennison E, Wyawahare P, Gilmour M, Sim D, Easther S, Robinson G. Recovery of bone turnover after alcohol withdrawal: a pilot study. *Osteoporosis International.* 2013;24(Suppl 1: S176).

[14] Sobral-Oliveira MB, Faintuch J, Guarita DR, Oliveira CP, Carrilho FJ. Nutritional profile of asymptomatic alcoholic patients. *Arquivos de gastroenterologia.* 2011 Apr-Jun;48(2):112-8. PubMed PMID: 21709952. Epub 2011/06/29. eng.

[15] Wilkens Knudsen A, Jensen JE, Nordgaard-Lassen I, Almdal T, Kondrup J, Becker U. Nutritional intake and status in persons with alcohol dependency: data from an outpatient treatment programme. *European journal of nutrition.* 2014 Oct;53(7):1483-92. PubMed PMID: 24442425. Epub 2014/01/21. eng.

[16] Gonzalez-Reimers E, Alvisa-Negrin J, Santolaria-Fernandez F, Candelaria Martin-Gonzalez M, Hernandez-Betancor I, Fernandez-Rodriguez CM, et al. Vitamin D and nutritional status are related to bone fractures in alcoholics. *Alcohol and alcoholism* (Oxford, Oxfordshire). 2011 Mar-Apr;46(2):148-55. PubMed PMID: 21248027. Epub 2011/01/21. eng.

[17] Cummings SR, Nevitt MC, Browner WS, Stone K, Fox KM, Ensrud KE, et al. Risk factors for hip fracture in white women. *Study of Osteoporotic Fractures Research Group. The New England journal of medicine.* 1995 Mar 23;332(12):767-73. PubMed PMID: 7862179. Epub 1995/03/23. eng.

[18] Macdonald HM. Alcohol and recommendations for bone health: should we still exercise caution? *The American journal of clinical nutrition.* 2009 Apr;89(4):999-1000. PubMed PMID: 19244377. Epub 2009/02/27. eng.

[19] Gavaler JS. Effects of alcohol on endocrine function in postmenopausal women: a review. *Journal of studies on alcohol.* 1985 Nov;46(6):495-516. PubMed PMID: 4087913. Epub 1985/11/01. eng.

[20] Felson DT, Zhang Y, Hannan MT, Kannel WB, Kiel DP. Alcohol intake and bone mineral density in elderly men and women. *The Framingham Study. American journal of epidemiology.* 1995 Sep 1;142(5):485-92. PubMed PMID: 7677127. Epub 1995/09/01. eng.

[21] Laitinen K, Valimaki M, Keto P. Bone mineral density measured by dual-energy X-ray absorptiometry in healthy Finnish women. *Calcified tissue international.* 1991 Apr;48(4):224-31. PubMed PMID: 2059873. Epub 1991/04/01. eng.

[22] Tucker KL, Jugdaohsingh R, Powell JJ, Qiao N, Hannan MT, Sripanyakorn S, et al. Effects of beer, wine, and liquor intakes on bone mineral density in older men and women. *The American journal of clinical nutrition.* 2009 Apr;89(4):1188-96. PubMed PMID: 19244365. Pubmed Central PMCID: PMC2667462. Epub 2009/02/27. eng.

[23] National Osteoporosis Society. Hyperparathyoridism and Osteoporosis UK [updated April 2013; cited 2014 21/10/2014]. Available from: <http://www.nos.org.uk/document.doc?id=1363>.

[24] Smalls AG, Kloppenborg PW, Njo KT, Knoben JM, Ruland CM. Alcohol-induced Cushingoid syndrome. *British medical journal.* 1976 Nov 27;2(6047):1298. PubMed PMID: 1000199. Pubmed Central PMCID: PMC1690039. Epub 1976/11/27. eng.

[25] Diamond T, Stiel D, Lunzer M, Wilkinson M, Roche J, Posen S. Osteoporosis and skeletal fractures in chronic liver disease. *Gut.* 1990 Jan;31(1):82-7. PubMed PMID: 2318434. Pubmed Central PMCID: PMC1378345. Epub 1990/01/01. eng.

[26] Hay JE. Osteoporosis in liver diseases and after liver transplantation. *Journal of hepatology.* 2003 Jun;38(6):856-65. PubMed PMID: 12763383. Epub 2003/05/24. eng.

[27] Holbrook TL, Barrett-Connor E. A prospective study of alcohol consumption and bone mineral density. *BMJ* (Clinical research ed). 1993 Jun 5;306(6891):1506-9. PubMed PMID: 8518677. Pubmed Central PMCID: PMC1677960. Epub 1993/06/05. eng.

[28] Wosje KS, Kalkwarf HJ. Bone density in relation to alcohol intake among men and women in the United States. Osteoporosis international : a journal established as result of cooperation between the European Foundation for Osteoporosis and the National Osteoporosis Foundation of the USA. 2007 Mar;18(3):391-400. PubMed PMID: 17091218. Epub 2006/11/09. eng.

[29] Berg KM, Kunins HV, Jackson JL, Nahvi S, Chaudhry A, Harris Jr KA, et al. Association Between Alcohol Consumption and Both Osteoporotic Fracture and Bone Density. *The American Journal of Medicine.* 2008 5//;121(5):406-18.

[30] Sritara C, Thakkinstian A, Ongphiphadhanakul B, Pornsuriyasak P, Warodomwichit D, Akrawichien T, et al. Work- and Travel-related Physical Activity and Alcohol Consumption: Relationship With Bone Mineral Density and Calcaneal Quantitative Ultrasonometry. *Journal of clinical densitometry: the official journal of the International Society for Clinical Densitometry.* 2014 May 28. PubMed PMID: 24878331. Epub 2014/06/01. Eng.

[31] Yin J, Winzenberg T, Quinn S, Giles G, Jones G. Beverage-specific alcohol intake and bone loss in older men and women: a longitudinal study. *European journal of clinical nutrition.* 2011 Apr;65(4):526-32. PubMed PMID: 21326269. Epub 2011/02/18. eng.

[32] Coulson CE, Williams LJ, Brennan SL, Berk M, Kotowicz MA, Lubman DI, et al. Alcohol consumption and body composition in a population-based sample of elderly Australian men. *Aging clinical and experimental research.* 2013 May;25(2):183-92. *PubMed PMID*: 23739904. Epub 2013/06/07. eng.

[33] Eleftheriou KI, Rawal JS, James LE, Payne JR, Loosemore M, Pennell DJ, et al. Bone structure and geometry in young men: the influence of smoking, alcohol intake and physical activity. *Bone.* 2013 Jan;52(1):17-26. PubMed PMID: 22985892. Epub 2012/09/19. eng.

[34] Fehily AM, Coles RJ, Evans WD, Elwood PC. Factors affecting bone density in young adults. *The American journal of clinical nutrition.* 1992 Sep;56(3):579-86. PubMed PMID: 1503072. Epub 1992/09/01. eng.

[35] Korkor AB, Eastwood D, Bretzmann C. Effects of gender, alcohol, smoking, and dairy consumption on bone mass in Wisconsin adolescents. WMJ: official publication of the State Medical Society of Wisconsin. 2009 Jul;108(4):181-8. PubMed PMID: 19753823. Epub 2009/09/17. eng.

[36] Winther A, Dennison E, Ahmed LA, Furberg AS, Grimnes G, Jorde R, et al. The Tromso Study: Fit Futures: a study of Norwegian adolescents' lifestyle and bone health. *Archives of osteoporosis.* 2014;9:185. PubMed PMID: 24893722. Epub 2014/06/05. eng.

[37] Lucas R, Fraga S, Ramos E, Barros H. Early initiation of smoking and alcohol drinking as a predictor of lower forearm bone mineral density in late adolescence: a cohort study

in girls. *PloS one.* 2012;7(10):e46940. PubMed PMID: 23094033. Pubmed Central PMCID: PMC3475705. Epub 2012/10/25. eng.

[38] Dorn LD, Beal SJ, Kalkwarf HJ, Pabst S, Noll JG, Susman EJ. Longitudinal impact of substance use and depressive symptoms on bone accrual among girls aged 11-19 years. The Journal of adolescent health: official publication of the Society for Adolescent Medicine. 2013 Apr;52(4):393-9. PubMed PMID: 23298983. Pubmed Central PMCID: PMC3608731. Epub 2013/01/10. eng.

[39] Khoo CC, Woo J, Leung PC, Kwok A, Kwok T. Determinants of bone mineral density in older postmenopausal Chinese women. *Climacteric: the journal of the International Menopause Society*. 2011 Jun;14(3):378-83. PubMed PMID: 21401441. Epub 2011/03/16. eng.

[40] Sommer I, Erkkila AT, Jarvinen R, Mursu J, Sirola J, Jurvelin JS, et al. Alcohol consumption and bone mineral density in elderly women. *Public health nutrition.* 2013 Apr;16(4):704-12. PubMed PMID: 22800300. Epub 2012/07/18. eng.

[41] McLernon DJ, Powell JJ, Jugdaohsingh R, Macdonald HM. Do lifestyle choices explain the effect of alcohol on bone mineral density in women around menopause? *The American journal of clinical nutrition.* 2012 May;95(5):1261-9. PubMed PMID: 22456655. Epub 2012/03/30. eng.

In: Bone Disorders, Screening and Treatment
Editor: Aubrey M. Stone

ISBN: 978-1-63482-155-1


Chapter 6

# Nutritional Rickets and Hypovitaminosis D in the Upper Midwest, USA

***Mark K. Huntington*, MD PhD FAAFP***
Director, Sioux Falls Family Medicine Residency Program
Center for Family Medicine, Sioux Falls, South Dakota
Professor, Department of Family Medicine
University of South Dakota Sanford School of Medicine,
Sioux Falls, South Dakota

## Abstract

The annual incidence of rickets in the United States is low, at approximately 0.5 per 100,000. This has been achieved largely through vitamin fortification of foodstuffs, primarily dairy products. However, in 2007 one academic primary care clinic located in the eastern portion of the state of South Dakota, whose patient population includes a high proportion of immigrants, experienced an incidence that was 200 times that level. Starting from a discussion of these cases, this chapter reviews the literature regarding rickets and hypovitaminosis D in the upper Midwest region. It discusses specific risks in this population, including environmental factors present in northern climates, physiological factors inherent in subsets of the population, and specific cultural factors, all of which exert significant influences on vitamin D levels and risk of rickets. Prevention, diagnosis, and treatment strategies are presented from the perspectives of primary care of the individual, population health, and public policy.

* Corresponding Address: Center for Family Medicine; 1115 East 20th Street, Sioux Falls, SD 57105 USA; 605.575.1642, fax 605.335.1006; mark.huntington@usd.edu.

# Introduction

Rickets, a condition in children most commonly resulting from vitamin D deficiency, has long been the bane of life in northern cities. The move indoors, coupled with the increased air pollution of the industrial revolution, decreased exposure to the sun's ultraviolet rays necessary for vitamin D synthesis led to a nearly ubiquitous condition of long bone deformities, curvature of the spine, "rosary" deformations of the bony thorax, and severe muscle weakness. Autopsy studies in the 1800s identified rickets in nearly 90% of children in the cities of Boston, USA, and Leiden, Netherlands [1].

In the United States, rickets was essentially eliminated as a significant public health problem during the 1930s, in large part through the voluntary supplementation of foodstuffs – primarily dairy products – with vitamin D. However, in more recent years there has been a resurgence of rickets [2, 3]. While cases in the southern parts of the nation have received the most attention [4-6], the problem is not restricted to these areas.

In 2007, our institution – an academic primary care clinic located in the eastern portion of the state of South Dakota – experienced an incidence of rickets that was 200 times the national incidence, including one fatality. This prompted a series of studies of the epidemiology of hypovitaminosis in our local area which helped to define the extent of the problem and direct the development of solutions [7-9]. The focus of this chapter is a review of the reports of rickets in the upper Midwest portion of the United States (Figure 1). We will summarize our experiences, as well as those in neighboring states, and integrate them to offer recommendations that are relevant clinically, and to public health and policy.

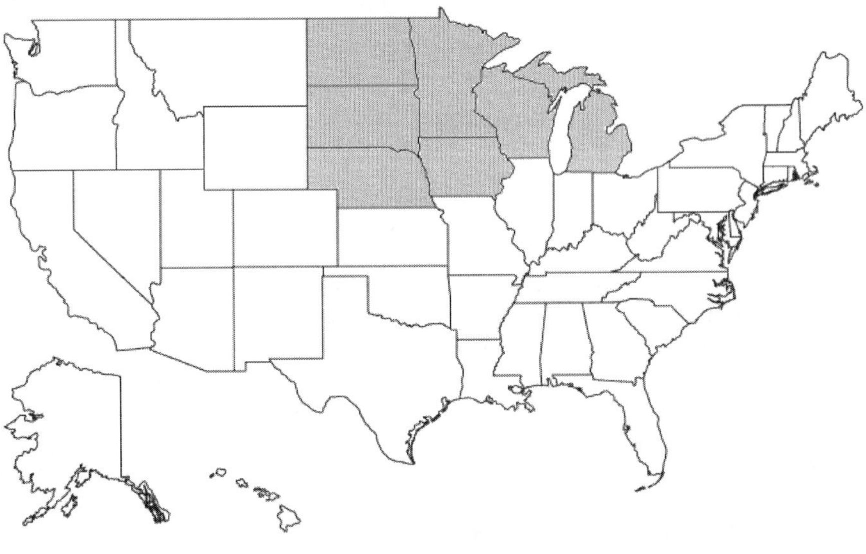

Figure 1. Shaded states are those whose rickets cases are discussed in this chapter.

# Methods

Literature searches were done on the PubMed database (www.ncbi.nlm.nih.gov/pubmed), employing terms "rickets", "hypovita-minosis", or "prevalence 'hypovitaminosis D'", each combined with the state name. State names included "Dakota", "Iowa", "Michigan", "Minnesota", "Nebraska", or "Wisconsin". Citation lists included in relevant papers identified via electronic search were reviewed in an attempt to identify any additional reports of potential interest in non-indexed publications (the "gray literature"). Research studies or case reports of non-human rickets were noted but excluded from this chapter. Similarly, the focus was limited to reports involving nutritional rickets; inherited conditions were excluded from the review. Articles on hypovitaminosis D addressing basic biomedical sciences or clinical implications and manifestations other than rickets were also excluded as beyond the scope of this chapter. General review articles originating from, but not specifically citing cases or epidemiological data in, the geographic area of interest were not included.

Studies retrieved reported serum 25-hydroxyvitamin D (calcidiol) levels in several ways; predominantly, the values were expressed as nanograms per milliliter (ng/mL). This chapter follows suite; to convert these values to nanomoles per liter (nmol/L), multiply by 2.5 (Table 1).

**Table 1. Conversion of units**

| Vitamin D levels: | | |
|---|---|---|
| | nmol/L = | ng/mL x 2.5 |
| | ng/mL = | $\frac{\text{nmol/L}}{2.5}$ |

# Results

Our literature search turned up relatively few relevant articles on human rickets in the upper Midwest (Table 2). Reports of veterinary rickets cases, case reports in which rickets was merely considered in the differential diagnosis or discussion, laboratory and clinical research papers, general review papers on the topic of rickets originating from institutions within the geographical area of interest, and papers addressing non-D hypovitaminosis composed the bulk of the publications identified.

## The Dakotas

No rickets case reports were retrieved for the Dakotas using our search strategy, including the one originating from our institution. The primary author on that report had relocated prior to its publication, thus was not associated with the state of South Dakota. Literature on the prevalence of hypovitaminosis D in the Dakotas indexed on PubMed was found to originate exclusively from our institution, though other publications relating hypovitaminosis D to other conditions originated from institutions in these states [10, 11].

**Table 2. Citations relevant to rickets in the upper Midwest retrieved via PubMed**

| | Total citations retrieved | Nutritional rickets case reports/case series | Vitamin D epidemiological studies** | Nonhuman rickets cases |
|---|---|---|---|---|
| (A) Search terms: "rickets" + state* | | | | |
| Dakota | 4 | 0 | 0 | 0 |
| Iowa | 10 | 0 | 0 | 5 |
| Michigan | 39 | 1 | 2 | 0 |
| Minnesota | 36 | 2 | 1 | 2 |
| Nebraska | 6 | 0 | 0 | 1 |
| Wisconsin | 48 | 1 | 1 | 3 |
| (B) Search terms: "hypovitaminosis" + state* | | | | |
| Dakota | 23 | 0 | 4 | 0 |
| Iowa | 105 | 0 | 2 | 5 |
| Michigan | 182 | 2 | 5 | 0 |
| Minnesota | 136 | 0 | 5 | 2 |
| Nebraska | 54 | 0 | 4 | 0 |
| Wisconsin | 269 | 1 | 5 | 3 |

* There was substantial – but not complete – overlap of the articles retrieved using the search strategies in (A) and (B).

** excluding non-rickets disease-association studies.

Following a case of severe rickets in an infant that resulted in death, a second case was identified in the same clinic (located at 44ºN) [12]. Physical, radiological, and laboratory findings were classic for rickets. The diagnosis was made based on the former, with the subsequent studies confirming the clinical impression. This child did well, and the case formed the basis for an educational "Grand Rounds" article on the diagnosis and treatment of rickets in the *Journal of Family Practice*. Several other rickets cases, including another which warranted publication, were also diagnosed in this clinic's population during this time [9].

The clinic to which these cases presented is the continuity clinic for a Family Medicine Residency Training program; among the population served are a large number of refugee immigrants [13]. Both cases were from the local population of refugees from the horn of Africa. As immigration from this region was ongoing, it raised the question regarding the vitamin D status of the new arrivals. A prospective study was undertaken, and identified that the vast majority (64-99%, depending on calcidiol level identified as 'normal') of new refugees were vitamin D deficient, some severely deficient [8]. This finding resulted in the institution of a policy to routinely replete all new refugees to ensure adequate levels. A subsequent study in the same portion of the state identified endemic hypovitaminosis in the adult population, regardless of refugee/immigrant status or degree of skin pigmentation [7]. The subpopulation of adults with the most pronounced hypovitaminosis D was that of pregnant women.

A study of American Indians children in South Dakota (43ºN), while focused primarily on the association of hypovitaminosis D with diabetes, found deficiency (<30 ng/mL) in 97% of the population, with the mean calcidiol level of 17 ng/mL (±8 ng/mL) [10]. No seasonal difference was noted in the prevalence of hypovitaminosis D; mean levels were lower in girls than boys ($p = 0.02$) and in teenagers than in elementary school aged children ($p = 0.002$).

No case reports of rickets or epidemiological studies of hypovitaminosis D were identified for North Dakota.

## Iowa

Although reports of veterinary rickets were identified, no human case reports originating from Iowa were found. However, two epidemiological studies of hypovitaminosis D in Iowa populations – which may serve as a proxy for risk of rickets – were retrieved.

A survey in the late 1980s looked at 373 women age 20-80, living in rural Iowa (42°N) [14]. Although the authors reported "low levels of calcidiol…were not observed", the mean was 24.1 ng/mL (±8 ng/mL). Today, values under 30 ng/mL are generally considered deficient. Twenty years later, at 41°N, a study of 35 breastfed infants (who were not receiving vitamin supplementation) found that 23% had levels less than 11 ng/mL, with nearly 6% below 5 ng/mL. Prevalence was greatest among dark-skinned infants, and was also markedly seasonal, with prevalence of deficiency rising to 78% in the winter.

## Minnesota

Over an 18-month period in the mid-1990s, 7 cases of nutritional rickets were diagnosed in the Twin Cities metropolitan area (45°N) [15]. In each case, the infants were exclusively breastfed without vitamin supplementation. Cases were diagnosed between 6 and 20 months of age, and all presented in the springtime following the long Minnesota winter. Two patients were described as "white", three as "black", one as "Iranian", and one as "mixed".

In 2013, a group of investigators at the Mayo Clinic undertook a retrospective study of the epidemiology of rickets in Olmsted County (44°N) [16]. They identified 17 children with nutritional rickets who were treated between 1970 and 2009. All rickets patients were younger than 3 years of age and 76% were described as "nonwhite", 59% as "black". In addition to race, nutritional rickets was associated with breastfeeding and poor growth. They identified a temporal trend, with the incidence of rickets increasing from 0 to 2.2 to 3.7 to 24.1 per 100,000 for the 1970s, 1980s, 1990s, and 2000s, respectively (incidence trend $p$ = 0.003).

Several reports of the epidemiology of hypovitaminosis D in Minnesota were identified, each having as its focus a specific subpopulation. No data on the overall population was found.

Refugees from sub-Saharan Africa have been the largest group immigrating to the Twin Cities in recent years. A retrospective study of the vitamin D status of adult patients in this population found that hypovitaminosis was significantly more prevalent than among US-born individuals (60% vs. 35.1%; $p < 0.001$), with severe deficiency – defined as < 10 ng/mL – showing a similar pattern (15.1% vs.7.9%; $p = 0.02$) [17]. A significant seasonal variation was noted, with highest vitamin D levels being found from June to August ($p < 0.001$).

In addition to refugees, the vitamin D status in immigrants of another sort has been investigated in Minnesota. A prospective cohort study at an international adoption clinic found that when tested within 6 months of adoption, 27% of children had insufficiency (<20 ng/mL) and 8% had deficiency (<8 ng/mL) [18]. No mention of clinical rickets was made.

In a study of the correlation between chronic pain and vitamin D deficiency, 93% of all patients – and 100% of patients of African-American, East African, Hispanic, and American Indian ancestry – had hypovitaminosis D (defined as <20 ng/mL) [19]. A seasonal variation of 3.5 ng/mL between mean levels in winter vs. summer was found. Levels in women of childbearing age were significantly lower than those of nonchildbearing age ($p < 0.001$). Levels for male and female patients was not different overall, but was significantly lower in female immigrants from East Africa than their male counterparts ($p < 0.001$). The authors did not investigate how these epidemiological findings in the chronic pain patient subpopulation compared to their patient population in general.

## Michigan

Several case series of rickets were identified originating from Michigan. A 1987 paper pointed out a resurgence of nutritional rickets that was noted in the contemporary pediatric literature, and added a contribution to the orthopedic literature of 3 cases [20]. Patients' age ranged from 14-17 months, all were African-American, and all were exclusively breastfed for an extended period. All patients recovered following simple vitamin D supplementation. A similar series of 4 cases composed a didactic review article a dozen years later [21]. Each of these cases was also African-American, ages 6-18 months, with a history of exclusive breastfeeding without vitamin supplementation.

A 10-year retrospective, single institution study performed at a Detroit (42ºN) children's hospital identified 58 nutritional rickets cases between 1995 and 2005 [22]. Patients were predominantly male (62%), ages 2-132 months, and mainly African-American (81%). Ninety-six percent were exclusively breast-fed without vitamin supplementation, and three-quarters of the cases occurred in the second half of the study period. The majority of cases presented via the emergency department (79%), and one-third of the patients were hospitalized. There was a seasonal predominance of cases, with 52% presenting in winter and spring and 14% in the summer.

Three epidemiological studies of the prevalence of hypovitaminosis D in Michigan were retrieved. A 2007 study of 96 uninsured women in urban Flint, MI (43°N) found deficiency, defined as <20 ng/mL, in 67% of women age 21-65 years of age [23]. Non-caucasians were three times more likely than Caucasians to be deficient. A subsequent study of Arab-American women in Dearborn, MI (43°N) found uniformly low vitamin D levels [24]. The authors compared veiled and unveiled women and found median calcidiol levels of 8.5 ng/mL in unveiled women, 7 ng/mL in veiled but vitamin D supplemented women, and 4 ng/mL in unveiled, unsupplemented women. The levels were significantly different between veiled and unveiled women ($p = 0.003$), but with supplementation of veiled women, this became insignificant ($p = 0.09$). Comparison with supplemented, unveiled women was not reported. Finally, a study of 2839 obstetrical patients in Detroit (42ºN) found 71.7% of women had deficiency (<20 ng/mL) [25]. The highest prevalence was in Arab-Americans (91.8%), African-Americans (81.6%), and Asian-Americans (74.3%). Women wearing the hijab ("veiled women" of the previously-cited study) were more likely to be deficient (89.5% vs. 68.7%, $p = 0.0001$).

### Nebraska

No rickets case reports or case series were identified from this state. A study of 1179 postmenopausal women in rural eastern Nebraska was undertaken to develop a picture of vitamin D status in this population [26]. Mean calcidiol level was 28.7 ng/mL (±8 ng/mL), with 68% of subjects falling below 32 ng/mL. There was a seasonal variation of 2.1 ng/mL, which was significant ($p = 0.001$). A case-control study of vitamin D status in pre-operative bariatric vs. non-obese patients found 90% of obese patients and 32% non-obese controls had calcidiol levels below 30 ng/mL [27]. Both these studies occurred at 41°N.

### Wisconsin

In one of the largest rickets case series published in the last half century, a 2004 single-institution review of inpatient and outpatient rickets diagnoses through Children's Hospital of Milwaukee – located at 43°N – identified 51 cases of nutritional rickets [28]. All were associated with breastfeeding in the absence of vitamin supplementation. Mean age at diagnosis was 13.6 months, and 90% of those diagnosed were African-American, despite the "comparatively low rate of breast feeding in African-Americans" in their patient population. The authors commented on the lack of availability of a vitamin D supplement for infants as a challenge to prevention and treatment of rickets. Additionally, they noted that 14% of those diagnosed with rickets in their study were identified incidentally, suggesting that asymptomatic, untreated rickets may be more widespread than recognized.

Subsequently, a study of 71 older women (mean age 76 years) identified hypovitaminosis D in 59% of them [29]. The authors of this study call for action to address "a Wisconsin epidemic", pointing out that though this study was of elderly women, the geographic and seasonal limits on cutaneous vitamin D biosynthesis place all of the state's residents at risk.

## Discussion

### Epidemiological Trends

Essentially all of the studies identified in this survey indicated high prevalence of hypovitaminosis D in the upper Midwest. Several of the studies indicate an increasing incidence of rickets (Figure 2). This apparent trend is concerning. The potential public health significance of this calls for efforts to interrupt this pattern. In developing a strategy to address the problem, an understanding of reason for this trend would be helpful.

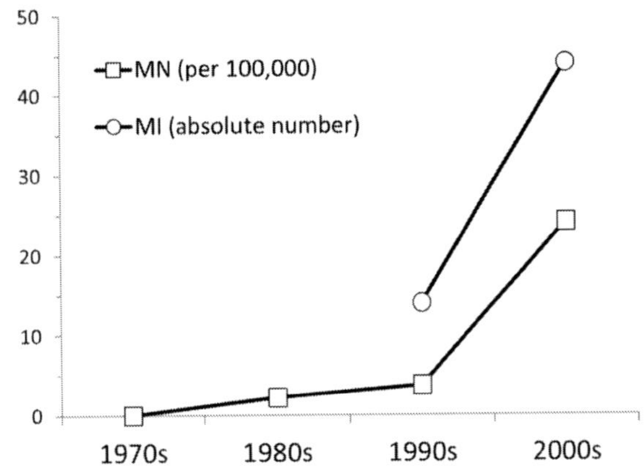


Figure 2. Changing epidemiology of rickets in the upper Midwest. Prevalence of rickets in a Minnesota study show an increase since the 1970s [16]; a Michigan case series demonstrates a similar pattern [22].

## Risk Factors

Nutritional rickets is the result of hypovitaminosis D. Risk of developing hypovitaminosis, and thus rickets, is dependent upon a number of factors. These include environmental conditions, physiological traits, cultural and behavioral characteristics, and perinatal conditions.

### *Environmental*

A seasonal variation in the incidence of rickets has long been recognized [30]. The shorter daylight hours, an increased proportion of time spent indoors, and the greater amount of clothing worn during the winter result in both decreased amounts of sunlight and decreased surface area exposed to it, which greatly decrease the amount of cutaneous vitamin D photosynthesis.

In addition, the angle of the sunlight passing through the atmosphere further diminishes the quantity of ultraviolet light reaching the individual, in a fashion dependent upon not only season but time of day and latitude [31]. Variations of cloud cover may contribute to this [32]. Cloud cover and airborne pollution levels are negatively correlated with effectiveness of cutaneous vitamin D synthesis [33-35]. Extensive investigations have characterized these changes in Boston, MA, (42°N) and Edmonton, AB, (52°N). Cutaneous photosynthesis of vitamin D was virtually nonexistent from November through February in the former, and Mid-October through April in the latter [36]. In contrast, photosynthesis continued throughout the year in Los Angeles, CA (34°N).

Located between 40°N (southern border of Nebraska) and 49°N (northern border of Minnesota), the upper Midwest is significantly affected by seasonal environmental factors that influence vitamin D levels. Several of the papers investigating hypovitaminosis D in this region measured the seasonal effect at approximately 3 ng/mL difference in mean serum levels between winter and summer [19, 26]. Seasonal variation in the Midwest, illustrated by two of the studies reviewed here, is shown in Figure 3.

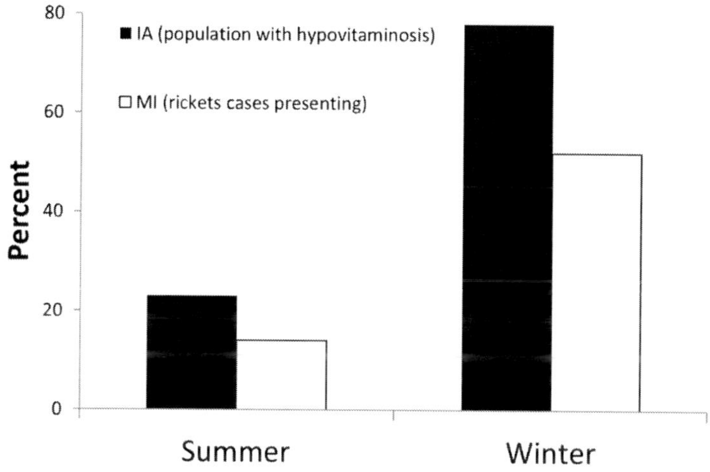


Figure 3. Seasonal differences. Percent of an Iowa study population with hypovitaminosis D and percent of rickets cases in a Michigan series presenting in each season.

### *Physiological*

Skin pigmentation levels have been long associated with lower vitamin D levels [37-39]. Investigations of vitamin D photosynthesis in humans demonstrate an inverse relationship between level of pigmentation and vitamin D conversion. *In vitro* studies showed a 6-fold increase in photosynthesis between dark and light skin in sunlight, and *in vivo* studies by the same investigators of volunteers on tanning beds found a 2-fold difference in increase of serum levels of calcidiol between dark and light skin [40]. Earlier studies found that light-skinned subjects had a serum calcidiol level increase of up to 60-fold over baseline when measured 24-48 hours after exposure to a single standardized dose of ultraviolet irradiation, while those with dark skin saw no significant change. Increasing the dose of the exposure given to those with dark skin six-fold resulted in changes similar to those seen following the standard dose in light-skinned subjects [39].

In the US, there has been a significant increase in immigration from Africa, alluded to in several of the reports on rickets and hypovitaminosis D in the upper Midwest. Census figures indicate there has been a doubling of immigration from Africa each decade (Figure 4) [41]. These immigrants are at increased risk, given the combination of their pigmentation level and the limited ultraviolet exposure available at the northern latitudes.

### *Cultural and Behavioral*

In addition to the environmental risk factors inherent in the upper Midwest, and the physiological risk factors presented in the degree of pigmentation in some of the subpopulations in whom rickets and hypovitaminosis D were identified in the studies cited above, there are cultural risk factors, as well. A study in Turkey identified a significant effect on serum calcidiol levels presented by choice of clothing [42]. Mean vitamin D levels in women wearing western clothing were 29.7 ng/mL, compared to those wearing traditional Islamic dress (covering whole body but leaving the hands and face exposed) which had mean concentrations of 21.1 ng/mL, significant at the $p < 0.05$ level. A study of the Saudi population identified high prevalence of hypovitaminosis D. This was especially noteworthy

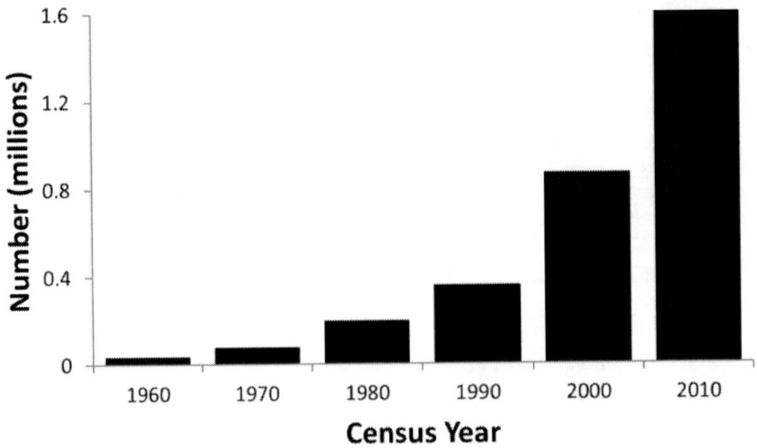


Figure 4. Foreign-born individuals from Africa residing in the United States (data from www.census.gov).

among women, of whom 35.6% had levels <10 ng/mL despite abundant sunshine [43]. This was a significantly higher prevalence than in men ($p < 0.0001$). Other investigators have found similar results, with the lowest calcidiol levels associated with the more conservative Islamic dress ($p < 0.001$) [44], though some authors point out the difficulty in separating clothing choice from overall nonexposure to the sun (i.e. indoor living) and a vitamin-deficient diet [45]. Several of the reports from the upper Midwest identify Muslim immigrants among those with very low serum vitamin D levels. While altering the culture, and thus deeply-held religious beliefs, may decrease the risk of hypovitaminosis D-related health issues, it is not necessarily a desirable intervention. However, an understanding of how culture affects risk may allow effective identification of candidates for more acceptable interventions such as dietary supplementation efforts.

Other cultural factors also may plan an important role in the risk of developing nutritional rickets. There has been a major change in behaviors over recent decades: the population is spending a greater proportion of its time indoors. Studies indicate that since the 1970s, children in both the US and UK spend 50% less time outside [46-49]. A variety of factors contribute to this, including increasing use of screen time (television, video games, internet), safety concerns, and lack of green space in which to play. This trend continues into adulthood, as well. From 1981-2005, there was a 25% decrease in overall outdoor recreational activities among Americans [50]. With an estimated 80-90% of city-dwellers' time spent indoors, there is limited opportunity for sun exposure and thus photosynthesis of vitamin D [51].

There have been changes in dietary culture in the US. Americans now drink 25% less milk than they did in 1975 (Figure 5) [52]. With dairy products representing a major source of dietary vitamin D, this is a potentially concerning trend. In a related vein, breastfeeding in the US has significantly increased, up from 25% in 1970s [53] to nearly 80% in 2013 (Figure 6) [54]. While overall this represents improved health practices and should not be discouraged, in the absence of supplementation risk of rickets is elevated [55-57].

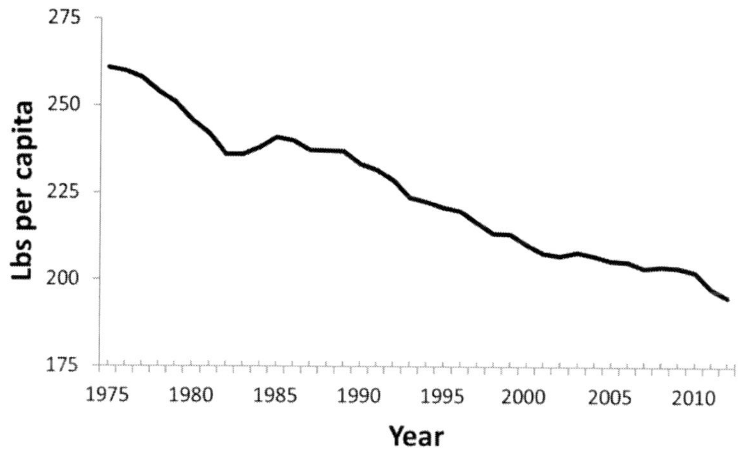


Figure 5. US annual per capita consumption of milk and cream (data from www.ers.usda.gov).

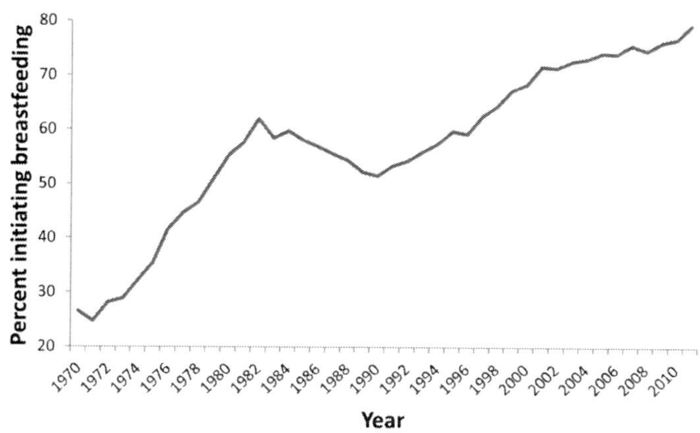


Figure 6. Percent of newborns in the US in whom breastfeeding is initiated. Data from Ross Mother's Surveys [58-60] and National Immunization Survey [61].

### *Perinatal*

Perhaps the greatest risk factor for nutritional hypocalcemic rickets is congenital. Although there exists a clinical entity of congenital rickets which develops prenatally in infants born to mothers with osteomalacia [62], here reference is made to something additional. Low maternal vitamin D stores – affected by all of the above risk factors – correlate to rickets risk in the infant through both low vitamin D reserves in the infant at birth and an even lower supply of vitamin D in the breast milk [62-70].

## Prevention

In considering the epidemiological data from the upper Midwest in context of the risk factors applicable to the subpopulations identified in the studies, there are several targeted interventions that should be considered in an effort to stem this re-emerging tide of nutritional rickets.

### Breastfeeding Infants

One recurring theme in the reports coming from the upper Midwest is the marked association between rickets and exclusive breastfeeding. An easy target for intervention is to supplement these infants with vitamin D. The American Academy of Pediatrics recommends that all infants (including those exclusively breastfed), children, and adolescents maintain a minimum daily intake of 400 IU of vitamin D [71]. This recommendation is largely evidence-based, and should be made to all expectant and newly-delivered mothers.

For some women, this recommendation may discourage them from breastfeeding their infants, as they may incorrectly conclude that breast milk is inferior to formula for infant health. For others, the recommended supplementation may be unacceptable as it is not "natural". In addition to these misperceptions, moving the preventative intervention further upstream may be desirable as it enhances maternal as well as child health.

### Pregnant Women

Ensuring that pregnant and nursing mothers have adequate vitamin D stores benefits maternal health and has the potential to reduce the incidence of rickets in infants. The subpopulation of adults with the most pronounced hypovitaminosis D in our South Dakota study was that of pregnant women [7]; other reports from the region also identified this subpopulation as being at risk [25]. This was especially significant, as low maternal vitamin D stores are associated with increased risk of rickets in breastfed infants. Some authors suggest that daily prenatal supplementation of 600-1000 IU and daily postpartum supplementation of 2000 IU may be effective at normalizing maternal vitamin D levels and reducing infant rickets risk [29, 64, 72]. While high quality studies of outcomes are lacking, there is some evidence in the literature indicating that ensuring that the nursing mother is vitamin D replete is comparable in terms of infant outcomes to supplementing the breastfed infant with the vitamin [72-74]. This is a low-risk intervention with the potential to make a significant difference.

### Refugee Immigrants

In addition to breastfed infants, another subpopulation identified as at risk for hypovitaminosis D and rickets are immigrants to the upper Midwest [75], likely related to low dietary intake, darker skin pigmentation, and a high level of clothing cover (for either religious reasons or for warmth in a climate far cooler than is found in their countries of origin). This represents an appropriate population to target for supplementation. Although a strong evidence base is lacking regarding the ideal dose for supplementation of refugees, 800-1000 IU daily has been suggested as a minimum [75]. In pursing this strategy, a variety of potential challenges must be kept in mind including health literacy, language, and economic barriers to its successful implementation [76].

An example of the latter challenge was encountered in South Dakota. In our newly-arrived refugee population, severe deficiency was prevalent enough that a policy was implemented to add routine supplementation to the initial new refugee medical evaluation, without testing serum calcidiol levels [8]. An initial barrier to the policy of vitamin D supplementation of newly-arriving refugees in the state was that vitamin D elixir was not on the drug formulary of the payer by whom the refugees were covered. The data from the study was cited to prompt a change in formulary to ensure the availability of an appropriate formulation for the youngest refugee children.

## Diagnosis

Although primary prevention of rickets is the best approach, it is imperfect. Some patients may fall through the cracks, and rickets will develop. Given its absence – until recently – from the limelight in clinical medicine in the Midwest, the diagnosis of rickets may be easily missed, leading to a delay in initiation of treatment. It is important for the region's clinicians to be diligent and maintain a high index of suspicion for rickets in at-risk populations.

### *Clinical Findings*

Often, early signs of rickets are rather nonspecific and include apathy, listlessness, and poor growth. There may be symptoms of neuromuscular dysfunction, including cramps, weakness with a waddling gait, hypotonia, numbness, paresthesias, tetany, and seizures. Skeletal findings include soft, misshapen head with widened sutures and frontal bossing, delayed eruption of teeth. Some of the skeletal findings that are more specific to rickets are the "rachitic rosary" (prominent costosternal joints), Harrison's groove (indentation at point of insertion of diaphragm, due to the pull of the diaphragm against the softened lower ribs), bowed limbs and other swollen joints. Maintaining a high degree of suspicion for children with identifiable risk factors is critical in ensuring timely diagnosis and treatment. When these clinical findings are present, use of ancillary diagnostic services can clarify and confirm the diagnosis.

### *Laboratory Investigation*

When rickets is suspected, appropriate laboratory evaluation should be performed. This includes excluding non-nutritional causes by checking creatinine and liver enzymes (normal value excludes renal insufficiency and liver disease as etiology). Serum phosphorus and parathyroid hormone (PTH) levels can aid in clarifying the diagnosis (normal phosphorus and PTH make rickets an unlikely diagnosis). Other findings found in nutritional rickets include elevated serum alkaline phosphatase and urinary phosphate levels, and decreased urine calcium levels and serum calcidiol levels. Often, serum calcium and calcitriol levels are normal.

### *Radiologic Findings*

Radiological findings generally establish the diagnosis. Epiphyses demonstrate widening and flaring with irregular "cupped" epiphyseal-metaphyseal junctions; involvement of the costrochondral junctions produces the rachitic rosary. Long bones are bowed ("sabre" shaped), with indistinct cortices, pathological fractures may be present, and pseudofractures (also called Looser's zone or Milkman's fractures) may be found on the concave side of clavicles, femoral neck, pubic rami, ribs, and on the lateral aspect of scapulae. Radiological studies were the means by which most of the "incidental" rickets cases were diagnosed in the Wisconsin study [28].

## Treatment

Asymptomatic, mild-to-moderate vitamin D deficiency can be corrected via supplementation as discussed above. Severe vitamin D deficiency and nutritional rickets generally requires more aggressive treatment, and may be remedied by replacement therapy anywhere along the vitamin D metabolic pathway.

The first option is administration of dihydrotachysterol (DHT; $D_1$), which is given as 60,000 IU once, then 6000 IU daily until the rickets are clinically and radiologically resolved. The next option is farther downstream: ergocalciferol ($D_2$) may be given as 1,000-5,000 IU daily for 6-12 weeks (1000 IU/day if age <1 month, 3000 IU/day if age 1-12 months, 5000 IU/day if over 12 months of age). A third treatment choice is at the final metabolic step: cholecalciferol ($D_3$, calcitriol). This is typically administered as either 5000-10,000 IU daily for 2-3 months. A final treatment option is stosstherapy, which may be especially valuable in cases when follow-up and multiple dosing can be a challenge due to logistics or noncompliance [77]. This consists of a bolus of cholecalciferol 150,000-600,000 IU given on a single day divided into 4-6 doses, or spread over several days for better tolerance (e.g. 300,000 IU over 1-7 days in children 1-12 months of age). Its onset of action is less than a day, with maximal effects seen in 4 weeks. Some preparations contain propylene glycol, which is limited to <25 mg/kg of body weight permissible in food additives due to potential toxicity. All of these vitamin D preparations have rather unpleasant tastes.

When possible, treatment of rickets should be monitored by checking serum calcium and alkaline phosphatase at one month, and serum calcium, magnesium, phosphate, alkaline phosphatase, calcidiol, PTH, and wrist x-ray at 3 months.

## Limitations

There are several limitations to this review. Few population-based studies were identified, with the majority of papers representing clinical case reports. The epidemiological publications identified focused primarily on specific subpopulations, thus the data and conclusions may not be applicable to the population as a whole. It is probable that some reports of rickets and hypovitaminosis D in the region of interest were missed by the literature search strategy. This certainly happened for one of the South Dakota papers to which the author of this chapter contributed [12]. The first-named author moved to different state prior to the paper's publication, and thus "Dakota" was not associated with the paper in the PubMed indexing.

# Conclusion

Both nutritional rickets and hypovitaminosis D are prevalent in the upper Midwest, and appear to be increasing. Important risk factors include latitude, climate, immigrant status, skin pigmentation, and cultural behaviors. Public health efforts at education and vitamin D supplementation specifically focused on infants, expectant and nursing mothers, and immigrants have the potential to decrease the risk of rickets in this region.

# References

[1] Holick MF. Resurrection of vitamin D deficiency and rickets. *J Clin Invest.* 2006;116(8):2062-72.

[2] Rowe PM. Why is rickets resurgent in the USA? *Lancet.* 2001;357(9262):1100.

[3] Weisberg P, Scanlon KS, Li R, Cogswell ME. Nutritional rickets among children in the United States: review of cases reported between 1986 and 2003. *Am J Clin Nutr.* 2004;80(6 Suppl):1697S-705S.

[4] Kreiter SR, Schwartz RP, Kirkman HN, Jr., Charlton PA, Calikoglu AS, Davenport ML. Nutritional rickets in African American breast-fed infants. *J Pediatr.* 2000;137(2):153-7.

[5] CDC. Severe malnutrition among young children--Georgia, January 1997-June 1999. *MMWR Morb Mortal Wkly Rep.* 2001;50(12):224-7.

[6] Tomashek KM, Nesby S, Scanlon KS, Cogswell ME, Powell KE, Parashar UD, et al. Nutritional rickets in Georgia. *Pediatrics.* 2001;107(4):E45.

[7] Bunde E, Hanssen K, Huntington MK. Vitamin D status in eastern South Dakota. *S D Med.* 2012;65(6):227, 9, 31.

[8] Huntington MK, Shafer CW, Pudwill R, Boer L, Kendall J. Prevalence of vitamin D deficiency among immigrants to South Dakota. *S D Med.* 2010;63(2):51-5.

[9] Elias AF, Dunn J, Huntington MK. Tuberculosis and profound hypovitaminosis D in an infant. *Pediatr Infect Dis J.* 2011;30(11):1008-10.

[10] Nsiah-Kumi PA, Erickson JM, Beals JL, Ogle EA, Whiting M, Brushbreaker C, et al. Vitamin D insufficiency is associated with diabetes risk in Native American children. *Clin Pediatr* (Phila). 2012;51(2):146-53.

[11] Senti J, Thiele DK, Anderson CM. Maternal vitamin D status as a critical determinant in gestational diabetes. *J Obstet Gynecol Neonatal Nurs.* 2012;41(3):328-38.

[12] Schmalz M, Boos K, Schmalz G, Huntington MK. Failure to thrive. *J Fam Pract.* 2009;58(10):539-44.

[13] Huntington MK, Shafer CW. The new South Dakotans: caring for recent immigrants. *S D Med.* 2008;61(11):409-15.

[14] Sowers MR, Wallace RB, Hollis BW, Lemke JH. Parameters related to 25-OH-D levels in a population-based study of women. *Am J Clin Nutr.* 1986;43(4):621-8.

[15] Eugster EA, Sane KS, Brown DM. Minnesota rickets. Need for a policy change to support vitamin D supplementation. *Minn Med.* 1996;79(8):29-32.

[16] Thacher TD, Fischer PR, Tebben PJ, Singh RJ, Cha SS, Maxson JA, et al. Increasing incidence of nutritional rickets: a population-based study in Olmsted County, Minnesota. *Mayo Clin Proc.* 2013;88(2):176-83.

[17] Campagna AM, Settgast AM, Walker PF, DeFor TA, Campagna EJ, Plotnikoff GA. Effect of country of origin, age, and body mass index on prevalence of vitamin D deficiency in a US immigrant and refugee population. *Mayo Clin Proc.* 2013;88(1):31-7.

[18] Gustafson KL, Eckerle JK, Howard CR, Andrews B, Polgreen LE. Prevalence of vitamin D deficiency in international adoptees within the first 6 months after adoption. *Clin Pediatr* (Phila). 2013;52(12):1149-53.

[19] Plotnikoff GA, Quigley JM. Prevalence of severe hypovitaminosis D in patients with persistent, nonspecific musculoskeletal pain. *Mayo Clin Proc.* 2003;78(12):1463-70.

[20] Kruger DM, Lyne ED, Kleerekoper M. Vitamin D deficiency rickets. A report on three cases. *Clin Orthop Relat Res.* 1987(224):277-83.

[21] Joiner TA, Foster C, Shope T. The many faces of vitamin D deficiency rickets. *Pediatr Rev.* 2000;21(9):296-302.

[22] Lazol JP, Cakan N, Kamat D. 10-year case review of nutritional rickets in Children's Hospital of Michigan. *Clin Pediatr* (Phila). 2008;47(4):379-84.

[23] Kakarala RR, Chandana SR, Harris SS, Kocharla LP, Dvorin E. Prevalence of vitamin D deficiency in uninsured women. *J Gen Intern Med.* 2007;22(8):1180-3.

[24] Hobbs RD, Habib Z, Alromaihi D, Idi L, Parikh N, Blocki F, et al. Severe vitamin D deficiency in Arab-American women living in Dearborn, Michigan. *Endocr Pract.* 2009;15(1):35-40.

[25] Collins-Fulea C, Klima K, Wegienka GR. Prevalence of low vitamin D levels in an urban midwestern obstetric practice. *J Midwifery Womens Health.* 2012;57(5):439-44.

[26] Lappe JM, Davies KM, Travers-Gustafson D, Heaney RP. Vitamin D status in a rural postmenopausal female population. *J Am Coll Nutr.* 2006;25(5):395-402.

[27] Goldner WS, Stoner JA, Thompson J, Taylor K, Larson L, Erickson J, et al. Prevalence of vitamin D insufficiency and deficiency in morbidly obese patients: a comparison with non-obese controls. *Obes Surg.* 2008;18(2):145-50.

[28] Mylott BM, Kump T, Bolton ML, Greenbaum LA. Rickets in the Dairy State. *WMJ.* 2004;103(5):84-7.

[29] Binkley N, Krueger D, Drezner MK. Low vitamin D status: time to recognize and correct a Wisconsin epidemic. *WMJ.* 2007;106(8):466-72.

[30] Kassowitz M. Tetanie und autointoxikation im kindesalter. *Wein Med Presse.* 1897;Nr 4/5.

[31] Holick MF. Environmental factors that influence the cutaneous production of vitamin D. *Am J Clin Nutr.* 1995;61(3 Suppl):638S-45S.

[32] Project ISCC. Seasonal Variations of Cloud and Surface Properties. Available from: http://isccp.giss.nasa.gov/climanal3.html.

[33] Parisi AV, Turnbull DJ, Downs NJ. Influence of high levels of cloud cover on vitamin D effective and erythemal solar UV irradiances. *Photochem Photobiol Sci.* 2012;11(12):1855-9.

[34] Grifoni D, Zipoli G, Sabatini F, Messeri G, Bacci L. Action spectra affect variability of the climatology of biologically effective ultraviolet radiation on cloud-free days. *Radiat Prot Dosimetry.* 2013;157(4):491-8.

[35] Engelsen O, Brustad M, Aksnes L, Lund E. Daily duration of vitamin D synthesis in human skin with relation to latitude, total ozone, altitude, ground cover, aerosols and cloud thickness. *Photochem Photobiol.* 2005;81(6):1287-90.

[36] Webb AR, Kline L, Holick MF. Influence of season and latitude on the cutaneous synthesis of vitamin D3: exposure to winter sunlight in Boston and Edmonton will not promote vitamin D3 synthesis in human skin. *J Clin Endocrinol Metab.* 1988;67(2):373-8.

[37] Bell NH, Greene A, Epstein S, Oexmann MJ, Shaw S, Shary J. Evidence for alteration of the vitamin D-endocrine system in blacks. *J Clin Invest.* 1985;76(2):470-3.

[38] Holick MF, MacLaughlin JA, Doppelt SH. Regulation of cutaneous previtamin D3 photosynthesis in man: skin pigment is not an essential regulator. *Science.* 1981;211(4482):590-3.

[39] Clemens TL, Adams JS, Henderson SL, Holick MF. Increased skin pigment reduces the capacity of skin to synthesise vitamin D3. *Lancet.* 1982;1(8263):74-6.

[40] Chen TC, Chimeh F, Lu Z, Mathieu J, Person KS, Zhang A, et al. Factors that influence the cutaneous synthesis and dietary sources of vitamin D. *Arch Biochem Biophys.* 2007;460(2):213-7.

[41] Gambino CP, Trevelyan EN, Fitzwater JT. *The Foreign-Born Population From Africa: 2008–2012.* Washington DC: US Department of Commerce, Economics and Statistics Administration US Census Bureau; 2014.

[42] Buyukuslu N, Esin K, Hizli H, Sunal N, Yigit P, Garipagaoglu M. Clothing preference affects vitamin D status of young women. *Nutr Res.* 2014;34(8):688-93.

[43] Hussain AN, Alkhenizan AH, El Shaker M, Raef H, Gabr A. Increasing trends and significance of hypovitaminosis D: a population-based study in the Kingdom of Saudi Arabia. *Arch Osteoporos.* 2014;9:190.

[44] Gannage-Yared MH, Chemali R, Yaacoub N, Halaby G. Hypovitaminosis D in a sunny country: relation to lifestyle and bone markers. *J Bone Miner Res.* 2000;15(9):1856-62.

[45] Al-Turki HA, Sadat-Ali M, Al-Elq AH, Al-Mulhim FA, Al-Ali AK. 25-Hydoxyvitamin D levels among healthy Saudi Arabian women. *Saudi Med J.* 2008;29(12):1765-8.

[46] Juster FT, Ono H, Stafford FP. Changing Times of American Youth: 1981-2003 Ann Arbor, MI: Institute for Social Research University of Michigan; 2004 [cited 2014 06 November]. Available from: http://ns.umich.edu/Releases/2004/Nov04/teen_time_report.pdf.

[47] Alliance_for_Childhood. The Loss of Children's Play: A Public Health Issue College Park, MD: Alliance for Childhood; 2010 [cited 2014 06 November]. Available from: http://www.habitot.org/museum/pdf/ play_research/Health_brief.pdf.

[48] Clements R. An Investigation of the status of outdoor play. *Contemporary Issues in Early Childhood.* 2004;5:68-80.

[49] National_Children's_Bureau. Unwelcoming communities stop children playing out 2013 [cited 2014 06 November]. Available from: http:// www.playday.org.uk/ media/media-releases/7-august-2013.aspx.

[50] Pergams ORW, Zaradic PA. Evidence for a fundamental and pervasive shift away from nature-based recreation. *Proceedings of the National Academy of Sciences.* 2008;105(7):2295-300.

[51] Jablonski NG, Chaplin G. Human skin pigmentation, migration and disease susceptibility. *Philos Trans R Soc Lond B Biol Sci.* 2012; 367(1590):785-92.

[52] Geuss J. Why does the US continue to drink less milk? 2013. Available from: http://www.dairyreporter.com/Commodities/Why-does-the-US-continue-to-drink-less-milk.

[53] Wright A, Schanler R. The resurgence of breastfeeding at the end of the second millennium. *J Nutr.* 2001;131(2):421S-5S.

[54] News C. Breast-feeding rates rise to 77 percent of U.S. moms 2013. Available from: http://www.cbsnews.com/news/cdc-breast-feeding-rates-rise-to-77-percent-of-us-moms/.

[55] Greer FR, Marshall S. Bone mineral content, serum vitamin D metabolite concentrations, and ultraviolet B light exposure in infants fed human milk with and without vitamin D2 supplements. *J Pediatr.* 1989;114(2):204-12.

[56] Hillman LS. Mineral and vitamin D adequacy in infants fed human milk or formula between 6 and 12 months of age. *J Pediatr.* 1990;117 (2 Pt 2): S134-42.

[57] Bly E, Huntington J, Harper AL. Clinical inquiry. What is the best age to start vitamin D supplementation to prevent rickets in breastfed newborns? Breastfed infants who take vitamin D beginning at 3 to 5 days of life don't develop rickets. *J Fam Pract.* 2013;62(12):755-63.

[58] Martinez GA, Nalezienski JP. The recent trend in breast-feeding. *Pediatrics.* 1979;64(5):686-92.

[59] Ryan AS. The resurgence of breastfeeding in the United States. *Pediatrics.* 1997;99(4):E12.

[60] Ryan AS, Wenjun Z, Acosta A. Breastfeeding continues to increase into the new millennium. *Pediatrics.* 2002;110(6):1103-9.

[61] CDC. National Immunization Survey 2013 [cited 2014 10 November 2014]. Available from: http://www.cdc.gov/breastfeeding/data/ NIS_data/index.htm.

[62] Teotia M, Teotia SP, Nath M. Metabolic studies in congenital vitamin D deficiency rickets. *Indian J Pediatr.* 1995;62(1):55-61.

[63] Pawley N, Bishop NJ. Prenatal and infant predictors of bone health: the influence of vitamin D. *Am J Clin Nutr.* 2004;80(6 Suppl):1748s-51s.

[64] Thandrayen K, Pettifor JM. Maternal vitamin D status: implications for the development of infantile nutritional rickets. *Rheum Dis Clin North Am.* 2012;38(1):61-79.

[65] Greer FR. 25-Hydroxyvitamin D: functional outcomes in infants and young children. *Am J Clin Nutr.* 2008;88(2):529S-33S.

[66] Thandrayen K, Pettifor JM. Maternal vitamin D status: implications for the development of infantile nutritional rickets. *Endocrinol Metab Clin North Am.* 2010;39(2):303-20, table of contents.

[67] AlFaleh KM, Al-Manie AM, Al-Mahmoud HF, Al-Razqan HM, Al-Mutlaq AB, Al-Rumaih SA, et al. Prevalence of vitamin D deficiency in Saudi newborns at a tertiary care center. *Saudi Med J.* 2014;35(2):178-82.

[68] Dawodu A, Tsang R. Vitamin D deficiency and rickets: possible role of maternal vitamin D deficiency. *Ann Trop Paediatr.* 2007;27(4):319.

[69] Salama MM, El-Sakka AS. Hypocalcemic seizures in breastfed infants with rickets secondary to severe maternal vitamin D deficiency. *Pak J Biol Sci.* 2010;13(9):437-42.

[70] Shenoy SD, Swift P, Cody D, Iqbal J. Maternal vitamin D deficiency, refractory neonatal hypocalcaemia, and nutritional rickets. *Arch Dis Child.* 2005;90(4):437-8.

[71] Wagner CL, Greer FR. Prevention of rickets and vitamin D deficiency in infants, children, and adolescents. *Pediatrics.* 2008;122(5):1142-52.

[72] Ala-Houhala M, Koskinen T, Terho A, Koivula T, Visakorpi J. Maternal compared with infant vitamin D supplementation. *Arch Dis Child.* 1986;61(12):1159-63.

[73] Haggerty LL. Maternal supplementation for prevention and treatment of vitamin D deficiency in exclusively breastfed infants. *Breastfeed Med.* 2011;6(3):137-44.

[74] Harvey NC, Holroyd C, Ntani G, Javaid K, Cooper P, Moon R, et al. Vitamin D supplementation in pregnancy: a systematic review. *Health Technol Assess.* 2014;18(45):1-190.

[75] Guigne F, Duke P, Rourke L. Is vitamin D deficiency an underreported issue in refugee health?: two cases of infants presenting with vitamin D-deficiency rickets. *Can Fam Physician.* 2013;59(6):641-3.

[76] Guigne F, Duke P, Rourke L. Looking beyond literacy: understanding and approaching barriers to refugee health in 2 cases of vitamin D-deficiency rickets. *Can Fam Physician.* 2013;59(6):607-8.

[77] Cesur Y, Caksen H, Gundem A, Kirimi E, Odabas D. Comparison of low and high dose of vitamin D treatment in nutritional vitamin D deficiency rickets. *J Pediatr Endocrinol Metab.* 2003;16(8):1105-9.

In: Bone Disorders, Screening and Treatment
Editor: Aubrey M. Stone

ISBN: 978-1-63482-155-1


*Chapter 7*

# Bone Fragility in Rickets

***Colin R. Paterson****
Formerly Department of Medicine, University of Dundee,
Dundee, Scotland

## Abstract

While the bone deformities classically associated with rickets have been recognised for many years, the fact that fractures also occur has been less well appreciated. In fact an association with fractures has been reported since the nineteenth century. This chapter summarises the published reports of fractures in rickets due to vitamin D deficiency. It is clear that fractures often occur spontaneously, may be asymptomatic and may be multiple. While the reported cases were identified because of the finding of radiological evidence of rickets it is important to recognise that rickets may occur without radiological abnormality. Fractures due to rickets are likely to be more frequent than the modest number of cases would suggest. The chapter reviews published reports on fracture risk associated with vitamin D deficiency. It also reviews fractures in forms of rickets not due to vitamin D deficiency and emphasises the differential diagnosis of fractures in young children.

## Introduction

Vitamin D deficiency is not at all uncommon worldwide, not least in developed countries [1-3]. The best known consequences for the skeleton are osteomalacia in adults and rickets in children. The clinical and radiological features of rickets have been well described for many years. The clinical features include bone pain and deformities including bow legs, knock knees, prominent costo-chondral junctions ('rachitic rosary') and enlargement of the bone ends. In the skull the anterior fontanelle may be large or persistent, there may be frontal

* Contact details: Dr Colin R Paterson, Temple Oxgates, Longforgan, Dundee DD2 5HS, Scotland. +44 1382 360240; c.s.paterson@btinternet.com.

bossing or craniotabes, palpable deformability of the skull vault under modest pressure. These classical deformities are not often seen in patients today.

Fractures and often multiple fractures have been reported in cases of rickets since at least 1883 [4-7]. As early as 1906 it was noted that the fractures were usually spontaneous and occurred without any history of trauma [5]. Recently a number of authors have suggested that fractures are very uncommon in rickets and that multiple fractures are not seen [8, 9]. This chapter explores the relationship of fractures to rickets and vitamin D deficiency. It also reports on fractures in types of rickets not thought to be caused by vitamin deficiency.

## Vitamin D Deficiency Rickets

In 1906 Dr Henry Feiss in Cleveland, Ohio reported a case of severe rickets in a four-year-old girl with marked knock knees, a rachitic rosary and a persistent anterior fontanelle. On radiology he found, to his surprise, three fractures of the arms "which I would have overlooked completely if the pictures had not been taken" [5].

In 1921 Park and Howland [6] in Baltimore reported 22 rachitic children aged between 8 months and 3½ years with deformities of the thorax. Most of the children also had multiple fractures of the extremities, often not recognised until examined radiologically. One child had 20 fractures. In 1938 Bevan [7] described a girl aged 26 months with rickets found to have 14 undisplaced spontaneous fractures of arms and legs and two clavicular fractures.

In a recent survey of case reports of fractures in rachitic children in the first two years of life 35 children were identified, 18 of whom had multiple fractures [10]. There were 58 diaphyseal fractures and at least 40 rib fractures. Most of these were undisplaced, most were asymptomatic and most were apparently spontaneous. The principal biochemical findings in this group of patients are summarised in Table 1.

**Table 1. Biochemical findings, when available, in 35 children with fractures and rickets thought to be due to vitamin D deficiency [10]**

| | Number of patients | Number abnormal | Percentage |
|---|---|---|---|
| Serum calcium < 8.8 mg/dL | 24 | 14 | 58 |
| Serum alkaline phosphatase high | 22 | 20 | 91 |
| Serum 25OHD < 10 ng/mL | 17 | 16 | 94 |
| Serum PTH raised | 10 | 10 | 100 |

Abbreviations: 25OHD: 25-hydroxyvitamin D. PTH: parathyroid hormone.
Conversion factors: Serum calcium: 1 mmol/L = 4 mg/dL.
Serum 25OHD: 1 ng/mL = 2.5 nmol/L.

Moon et al. [11] summarised the presentation in children with rickets in 17 series published since 2000. In all they identified 71 children whose rickets presented with fractures, 6 percent of those whose reason for presentation was reported.

In a study from Seattle Chapman et al. [12] undertook a retrospective review of radiographs of 40 children aged less than two years with radiological evidence of rickets.

They found seven with fractures including five with more than one. All the fracture patients were thought to have had nutritional rickets. The number of fractures is likely to be an underestimate since the extent of the radiological surveys was limited.

In a large study of Qatari children the fracture rates in 129 found to have rickets was compared with 411 without [13]. In the rachitic group the lifetime history of fractures (22.5%) was significantly more common than in the controls (13.5%).

While it is clear that fractures and often multiple fractures do occur in rickets (Figure 1) it should be noted that these reports are based only on patients with overt radiological evidence of rickets. It should be noted that radiological changes are seen only in a minority of children with significant vitamin D deficiency. For example Root et al. [14] described a boy of 13 months in Florida with severe hypocalcaemia and undetectable serum 25-hydroxyvitamin D (25OHD) who had no radiological signs of rickets in repeated skeletal surveys. Similarly in a group of infants with deficiency severe enough to cause hypocalcaemia and seizures one third had no radiological abnormalities [15]. This limitation of radiology is particularly true of children under the age of one year [2, 16, 17]. Histological evidence of rickets is often present in the absence of radiological abnormalities [18-20]. It is likely that fractures due to rickets are more frequent than the number of reported cases would suggest.

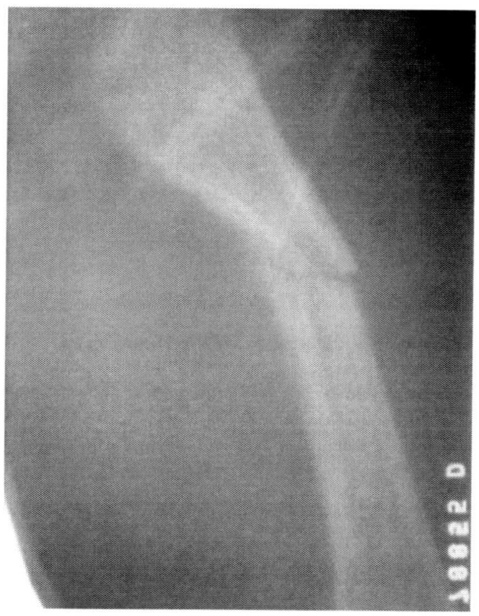

Figure 1. Oblique fracture of left femur in a boy aged 4 months. There was widespread evidence of rickets elsewhere in the skeleton. His family had a lifestyle that made vitamin D deficiency likely.

# Vitamin D Deficiency and Fractures

Several studies have explored the apparent risk of fractures in children said to have low levels of serum 25OHD. One difficulty in this field is the lack of consensus on what level is likely to reflect clinically significant deficiency and require treatment. Figures as low as 10ng/mL or as high as 40 ng/mL have been advocated [21, 22]. Most cases of rickets have levels lower than 10 ng/mL but there is some evidence that levels between 10 ng/mL and 20 ng/mL may be associated with increases in serum parathyroid hormone levels and with increased fracture risk in adults.

One relevant study was conducted by Perez-Rossello et al. [8]. They reported 40 children aged between eight months and two years said to have vitamin D deficiency. None was reported to have any fractures in response to a mailed questionnaire. However only two of their infants had any radiological features to suggest rickets. The remaining 38 children had a *median* serum 25OHD of 17ng/mL and normal serum parathyroid hormone levels. These children almost certainly had no significant deficiency and it seems unhelpful to regard the lack of fractures in the two who did as evidence against increased fracture risk in rickets. Others have outlined further difficulties with this study [23, 24].

Schilling et al. [25] described a study of 118 children aged less than two years with fractures. Only 8% of them had a serum 25OHD of less than 20 ng/mL. No information was provided on the number of children with serum 25OHD values less than 10 ng/mL. None of the children had radiological evidence of rickets. The authors found that there was no difference in the 25OHD levels between the children whose fractures were thought to have been caused by abuse and those not thought to have been abused. They concluded that vitamin D deficiency was unlikely to have played a part in the fractures. This conclusion is hard to justify with the small number of children who had significant deficiency. In addition there is a difficulty with the logic. One of the criteria for identifying abuse was the failure of the parents to explain the fractures. This is a characteristic feature of fractures associated with bone disorders including rickets [26] so that any rachitic patients might well be included in the 'abused' group. Other difficulties with this study are summarised elsewhere [27].

Similar concerns relate to a study by Contreras et al. [28]. They recruited 100 children with fractures aged under 18 years and 100 control subjects. They found no difference in serum 25OHD levels in the two groups or in the incidence of levels regarded as 'sufficient' (>30ng/mL), 'insufficient' (20-30 ng/mL) and 'deficient' (<20ng/mL). However only 20 of the 'fracture' cases had serum 25OHD levels less than 20 ng/mL and no information was provided on the number with levels lower than 10ng/mL. In addition the fracture and control groups were dissimilar; the fracture group was predominantly male. This study cannot be held to support the authors' view that vitamin D deficiency did not contribute to fracture risk.

One further study should be mentioned. Ryan et al. [29] examined bone mineral density and serum 25OHD levels in 76 African American children aged 5-9 years with forearm fractures. The values in these patients were compared with age-matched controls. The proportion of patients with a serum 25OHD less than 20 ng/mL was 47.1% compared with 40.9% for the controls. This difference was not significant but in a multivariate analysis it was found that the adjusted odds ratio was 3.46 (95% confidence intervals 1.09-10.94). The fracture patients also had lower Z-scores for bone mineral density. These results in a population in which vitamin D deficiency was not uncommon are consistent with a relationship to fracture risk.

## Pseudofractures

Both in adults with osteomalacia and in children with rickets fracture-like anomalies may be seen. These are known as pseudofractures or Looser zones or Milkman fractures. An example is shown in figure 2. It is often difficult to be sure whether an abnormality is a pseudofracture or a true fracture; the radiology may be very similar. One useful feature of a pseudofracture is the lack of local physical signs on clinical examination; histologically there is no discontinuity. A second notable feature of pseudofractures is the lack of the progressive radiological changes that would be expected of a fracture.

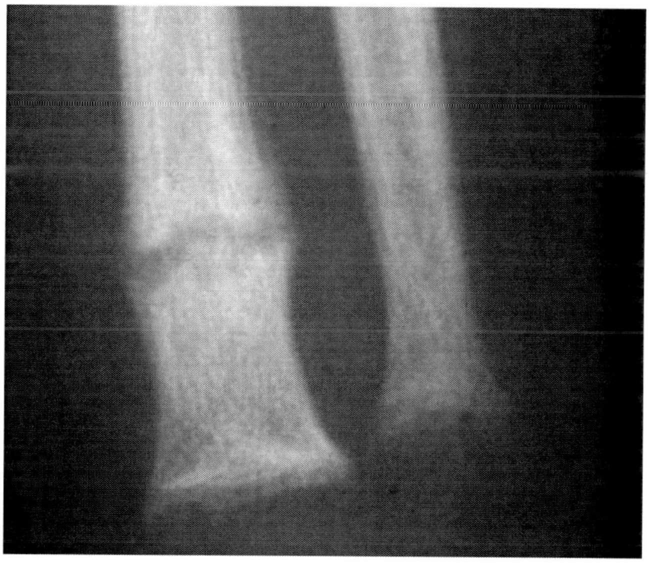

Figure 2. Pseudofracture of distal radius in an Asian boy aged 30 months.

## Other Forms of Rickets

### Osteopathy of Prematurity

This disorder is often called rickets but there is no evidence that vitamin D deficiency is responsible in most cases. Spontaneous fractures have been recognised for many years [30, 31] and often occur while a child is in a premature baby unit. Fractures include diaphyseal fractures (Figure 3), rib fractures (Figure 4) and metaphyseal lesions. Osteopenia is common but this is a very inexact assessment. Formal densitometry may be helpful in the future but at present interpretation is hampered by the lack of reference ranges. Biochemically many patients have raised values for serum alkaline phosphatase.

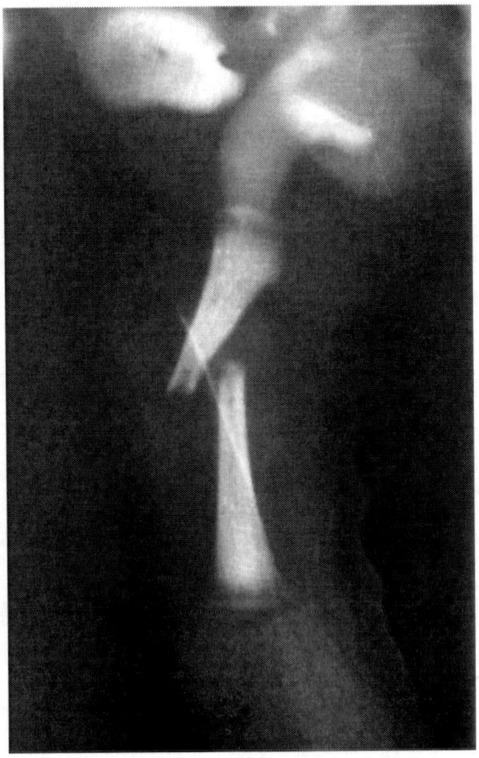

Figure 3. Fracture of right femur identified immediately after birth in a boy born at 31 weeks gestation by emergency caesarian section. Three weeks later while still in hospital five spontaneous rib fractures were found.

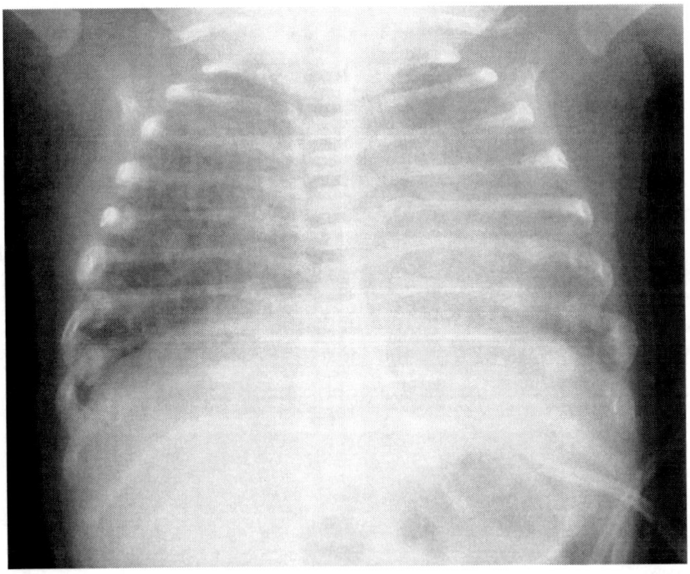

Figure 4. Multiple rib fractures in an 11 week old girl who had been born at 28 weeks gestation. All the fractures had occurred while she was in hospital.

## Hypophosphataemic Rickets

Rickets-like abnormalities are seen in a large number of disorders, mainly heritable, in which the major cause is hypophosphataemia due to impairment of phosphate reabsorption in the renal tubules. The best known of these is X-linked hypophosphataemia (vitamin D resistant rickets) but other heritable conditions have autosomal dominant or autosomal recessive inheritance [9]. In addition similar biochemical and clinical findings occur with benign tumours that secrete fibroblast growth factor 23 (tumour-induced osteomalacia) [32]. Fractures and pseudofractures do occur in adults with these disorders [33-35]. In one the patient had had fractures from the age of 14 [33]. One 11 year old boy with tumour-induced osteomalacia presented with a fractured femur [36].

## Antacid-induced Rickets

A special form of hypophosphataemic rickets has been described recently [37]. This results from the prolonged use of antacids containing aluminium hydroxide, which binds phosphate in the gut and so prevents its absorption. The resulting metabolic bone disease probably results not only from the hypophosphataemia but also from the aluminium, which has direct actions on bone. Multiple spontaneous fractures of ribs and long bones have been described in an 8-month old child who had received antacid for the preceding six months [38].

# Discussion

The fractures in rickets, like those in many other bone disorders (Paterson review), are often spontaneous and often asymptomatic. As with the other causes fractures found in young children may lead to the suggestion of non-accidental injury as the cause. There are published reports of this difficulty in children with rickets [2, 39, 40]. The small number of reported cases may be a serious underestimate. We know that even in western countries vitamin D deficiency is widespread. We know that the diagnosis of rickets may be difficult particularly in infants aged less than one year since radiological abnormalities are not consistently seen. It is important, therefore, to include vitamin D deficiency in the differential diagnosis of unexplained fractures in childhood.

One factor that plays a substantial part in current thinking is the view that metaphyseal fractures are specific pointers to non-accidental injury [41]. These are almost always asymptomatic and are found only with skeletal surveys, which are seldom justifiable except in children suspected of having been abused. While they were originally thought to represent traumatic avulsion of small fragments of bone and cartilage, this is now uncertain and they are often described as ‘metaphyseal lesions’ [42].

It is now clear that metaphyseal lesions have a substantial differential diagnosis including osteogenesis imperfecta, osteopathy of prematurity, hyperparathyroidism copper deficiency, Menkes’ syndrome and scurvy [26]. They may occur in infants with congenital neurological disorders, after ‘easy’ cesarean sections, after physiotherapy and in neonatal intensive care units [26]. In addition it has been noted that these lesions often resemble the metaphyseal changes of rickets, particularly healing rickets [42, 43]. It is clear that the certainties of the past on the nature of these lesions are no longer tenable. Cases of unexplained fractures of all sorts need to be investigated with an open mind.

## Acknowledgments

I am indebted to Dr. David Ayoub for drawing my attention to many of the articles cited here, to Mrs Sally Paterson for excellent help and to Dr Baoquiang Gao for the translation of reference 18.

## References

[1] Holick MF, Chen TC. Vitamin D deficiency; a worldwide problem with health consequences *Am J Clin Nutr* 2008; 87 (suppl): 1080S–6S.
[2] Keller KA, Barnes PD. Rickets vs. abuse: a national and international epidemic. *Pediatr Radiol* 2008; 38: 1210-6.
[3] Palacios C, Gonzalez L. Is vitamin D deficiency a major global public health problem? *J Steroid Biochem Mol Biol* 2014; 144A: 138-45.
[4] Meigs JF, Pepper W. *A Practical Treatise on the Diseases of Children.* (1883) Philadelphia: Blackiston .
[5] Feiss HO. Spontaneous fractures with rickets: report of a case. *J Bone Joint Surg Am* 1906; S2-3: 271-8.
[6] Park EA, Howland J. The dangers to life of severe involvement of the thorax in rickets. *Bull Johns Hopkins Hosp* 1921; 32:101-9 .
[7] Bevan R. Severe rickets with multiple spontaneous fractures. *Proc R Soc Med* 1938; 31: 361-4.
[8] Perez-Rossello JM, Feldman HA, Kleinman PK et al. Rachitic changes, demineralization and fracture risk in healthy infants and toddlers with a vitamin D deficiency. *Radiology* 2012; 262: 234-41.
[9] Elder CJ, Bishop NJ. Rickets. *Lancet* 2014; 383: 1665-76.
[10] Paterson CR. Fractures in rickets due to vitamin D deficiency. *Curr Orthop Pract* (in press).
[11] Moon RJ, Harvey NC, Davies JH, Cooper C. Vitamin D and skeletal health in infancy and childhood. *Osteoparos Int* 2014; 25: 2673-84.
[12] Chapman T, Sugar N, Done S, Marasigan J, Wambold N, Feldman K. Fractures in infants and toddlers with rickets. *Pediatr Radiol* 2010; 40:1184-9.
[13] Bener A, Al-Ali M, Hoffmann GF. Vitamin D deficiency in healthy children in a sunny country: associated factors. *Int J Food Sci Nutr* 2009; 60 suppl 5: 60-70.
[14] Root AW, Vargas A, Duckett GE, Hough G. Hypocalcaemia and hypovitaminosis D in an infant from Florida, the sunshine state. *J Fla Med Assoc* 1980; 67: 933-4.

[15] Ahmed I, Atiq M, Iqbal J, Khurshid M, Whittaker P. Vitamin D deficiency rickets in breast fed infants presenting with hypocalcaemic seizures. *Acta Paediatr* 1995; 84: 941-2.
[16] Wharton B, Bishop N. Rickets. *Lancet* 2003; 362: 1389-400.
[17] Pettifor JM, Isdale JM, Sahakian J, Hansen JDL. Diagnosis of subclinical rickets. *Arch Dis Child* 1980; 55: 155-7.
[18] Liu D. Pathological and X-ray study on bony specimens of rickets from 124 fetal and infantile autopsies. *Zhonghua Yi Xue Za Zhi* 1991; 71: 385-7.
[19] Cohen MC, Offiah A, Sprigg A, Al-Adnani M. Vitamin D deficiency and unexpected sudden death in infancy and childhood: a cohort study. *Pediatr Dev Pathol* 2013; 16: 292-300.
[20] Scheinberg I, Perry L. Does low vitamin D have a role in pediatric morbidity and mortality? An observational study of vitamin D in a cohort of 52 postmortem examinations. *Pediatr Dev Pathol* 2014; DOI: 10.2350/14-05-1491-OA.
[21] Shaw NJ, Mughal MZ. Vitamin D and child health: part 2 (extraskeletal and other aspects). *Arch Dis Child* 2013; 98: 368-72.
[22] Hollis BW, Wagner CL. Vitamin D requirements and supplementation during pregnancy. *Curr Opin Endocrinol Diabetes Obes* 2011;18: 371-5.
[23] Ayoub D. Fractures: abuse or rickets? *Radiology* 2012; 264: 614-5.
[24] Hyman C J. Fractures: abuse or rickets? *Radiology* 2012; 264: 615.
[25] Schilling S, Wood JN, Levine MA, Langdon D, Christian CW. Vitamin D status in abused and nonabused children younger than 2 years old with fractures. *Pediatrics* 2011; 127: 835-41.
[26] Paterson CR. Bone disease and fractures in early childhood. In *Child Abuse* (2012) ed Turner R A, Rogers H O, New York: Nova.
[27] Paterson CR. Vitamin D deficiency and fractures in childhood. *Pediatrics* 2011; 127: 973-4.
[28] Contreras JJ, Hiestand B, O'Neill JC, Schwartz R, Nadkarni M. Vitamin D deficiency in children with fractures. *Pediatr Emer Care* 2014; 30: 777-81.
[29] Ryan LM, Teach SJ, Singer SA et al. Bone mineral density and vitamin D status among African American children with forearm fractures. *Pediatrics* 2012; 130: e553-60.
[30] Dabezies EJ, Warren PD. Fractures in very low birth weight infants with rickets. *Clin Orthop Rel Res* 1997; 335: 233-9.
[31] Lucas-Herald A, Butler S, Mactier H, McDevitt H, Young D, Ahmed SF. Prevalence and characteristics of rib fractures in ex-preterm infants. *Pediatrics* 2012; 130: 1116-9.
[32] Jiang Y, Xia WB, Xing XP et al. Tumor-induced osteomalacia: an important cause of adult-onset hypophosphatemic osteomalacia in China: report of 39 cases and review of the literature. *J Bone Miner Res* 2012; 27: 1967-75.
[33] Baidya A, Chowdhury S, Mukhopadhyay S, Ghosh S. Hypophosphatemic rickets: a case of recurrent pathological fractures. *Indian J Endocrinol Metab* 2012; 16 (Suppl 2): S402-4.
[34] Tournis S, Koromila T, Chatzistamatas N et al. Hip fracture leading to the diagnosis of autosomal dominant hypophosphatemic rickets. *J Musculoskelet Neuronal Interact* 2013; 13: 391-4.

[35] Pahl DW, Kim CK. Bilateral femoral insufficiency fractures presenting as knee pain in a patient with hypophosphatemic vitamin D-resistant rickets. *Am J Orthop* 2008; 37: 315-7.

[36] Shulman DI, Hahn G, Benator R et al. Tumor-induced rickets: usefulness of MR gradient echo recall imaging for tumor localization. *J Pediatr* 2004; 144: 381-5.

[37] Chesney RW. A new form of rickets during infancy: phosphate depletion-induced osteopenia due to antacid ingestion. *Arch Pediatr Adolesc Med* 1998; 152: 1168-9.

[38] Robinson RF, Casavant MJ, Nahata MC, Mahan JD. Metabolic bone disease after chronic antacid administration in an infant. *Ann Pharmacother* 2004; 38: 265-8.

[39] Paterson CR. Vitamin D deficiency rickets and allegations of non-accidental injury. *Acta Paediatr* 2009; 98: 2008-12.

[40] Metz JB, Schwartz KA, Feldman KW, Lindberg DM. Non-cutaneous conditions clinicians might mistake for abuse. *Arch Dis Child* 2014; 99: 817-23.

[41] Ablin DS, Greenspan A, Reinhart M, Grix A. Differentiation of child abuse from osteogenesis imperfecta. *AJR Am J Roentgenol* 1990; 154: 1035-46.

[42] Offiah A, Van Rijn RR, Perez-Rossello JM, Kleinman PK. Skeletal imaging of child abuse (non-accidental injury). *Pediatr Radiol* 2009; 39: 461-70.

[43] Ayoub DM, Hyman C, Cohen M, Miller M. A critical review of the classic metaphyseal lesion: traumatic or metabolic? *AJR Am J Roentgenol* 2014; 202: 185-96.

In: Bone Disorders, Screening and Treatment
Editor: Aubrey M. Stone
ISBN: 978-1-63482-155-1


*Chapter 8*

# Diagnostic Strategies in Osteomalacia

***Colin R Paterson****

Formerly of Department of Medicine, University of Dundee, Dundee, Scotland

## Abstract

Many adults with osteomalacia due to vitamin D deficiency have symptoms for which the underlying cause may not be recognised for months or years. This chapter illustrates the clinical presentations including bone pain, muscle weakness and fractures. It summarises the investigative strategies that are appropriate. It covers the place of clinical examination, of biochemistry, of radiology, of densitometry and of bone biopsy. It also considers the rarer causes of osteomalacia including heritable forms of hypophosphataemia and tumour-induced osteomalacia (oncogenic osteomalacia).

## Introduction

Rickets in children and osteomalacia in adults have long been recognised as the bone disorders resulting from vitamin D deficiency. That they were essentially the same disorder was indicated by the fact that children with evidence of rickets at birth often had mothers with good evidence of osteomalacia [1]. Rickets and osteomalacia have similar histological findings with large amounts of uncalcified bone (osteoid). Apart from vitamin D deficiency similar histological and radiological findings are seen in less common metabolic disorders, particularly those charecterised by hypophosphataemia.

Vitamin D deficiency remains common worldwide [2,3]. The dietary sources of vitamin D are limited. It is most abundant in oily fish such as salmon, sardines and herring. Eggs are

* Corresponding author: Dr. Colin R Paterson, Temple Oxgates, Longforgan, Dundee DD2 5HS, Scotland, +44 1382 360240, c.s.paterson@btinternet.com.

sometimes a valuable source; their content depends on the diet of the hens and their exposure to sunlight. For most people, however, the principal source of vitamin D is its synthesis in the skin from 7-dehydrocholesterol in the presence of ultraviolet B (UVB) radiation. Despite the limitations of the climate most people in the UK obtain most of their vitamin D from exposure to sunlight. There are, however, substantial differences between individuals because of variations in lifestyle, skin pigmentation, clothing worn for cultural reasons and sunscreens. In addition UVB is attenuated at higher latitudes and by atmospheric pollution [4].

It is important to recognise that vitamin D is stored in adipose tissue for considerable periods. A person who is vitamin D replete may have sufficient stored vitamin D to last for two or more years. For example adults who in the past developed osteomalacia after partial gastrectomy only developed symptoms after several years [5]. In the management both of adults and of children with vitamin D deficiency single large doses may treat the disorder and prevent recurrence for many months [6].

Osteomalacia is well recognised as a consequence of malabsorption and may be the cause of the presenting symptoms. Coeliac disease, Crohn's disease, cystic fibrosis and primary biliary cirrhosis may lead to osteomalacia. Osteomalacia is recognised as a sequel to partial gastrectomy and to jejuno-ileal bypass surgery for obesity [7].

Apart from vitamin D deficiency osteomalacia is recognised as a consequence of hypophosphataemia, usually the result of renal tubular defects. Some of these disorders are heritable and include familial hypophosphataemia, inherited as a sex-linked dominant trait, and autosomal dominant hypophosphataemia. Others present sporadically; these include oncogenic osteomalacia caused by benign mesenchymal tumours that secrete fibroblast growth factor 23 (FGF23), which affects tubular phosphate reabsorption [8,9]. Hypophosphataemic osteomalacia has also been described as a consequence of long-term treatment with adefovir for hepatitis B [10].

## Presenting Symptoms

The classical presenting symptoms of osteomalacia are bone pain and muscle weakness; either may be the dominant complaint. The lack of specificity of these symptoms often means that patients remain without a correct diagnosis for months or years [11]. Many of the women whose osteomalacia was discovered after the birth of a rachitic child had already had symptoms for long periods. Similarly many patients with oncogenic osteomalacia have had symptoms of bone pain for years [8].

The bone pain may be misinterpreted. For example in patients with rheumatoid arthritis or osteoarthritis increasing pain may be attributed to deterioration in the underlying condition and treated inappropriately. In one study in the west of Scotland [12] the authors commented that osteomalacia is 'a common, easily overlooked and treatable cause of morbidity in elderly patients with rheumatoid arthritis'. Patients formally diagnosed as having fibromyalgia may similarly be found to have vitamin D deficiency [13].

The muscle weakness is typically a proximal myopathy and causes difficulty in climbing stairs or getting out of a chair.

Less commonly osteomalacia, like rickets, presents with fractures [14]. Any type of fracture may occur including fractures conventionally thought to represent osteoporosis, fractures of hips, vertebrae or distal forearm. Fractures may be spontaneous or occur with little recognised force (figure 1). Delay in fracture healing may be the first indication that the underlying cause was vitamin D deficiency [15]. In some parts of the world osteomalacia or previous osteomalacia may be the cause of pelvic deformity and obstructed labour [16].

Some patients with osteomalacia are asymptomatic and only identified after the finding of a low bone density (Table 1). It is important to recognise that a low bone density has a differential diagnosis. Some patients with undoubted osteomalacia, however, have bone density figures within the reference range (see below).

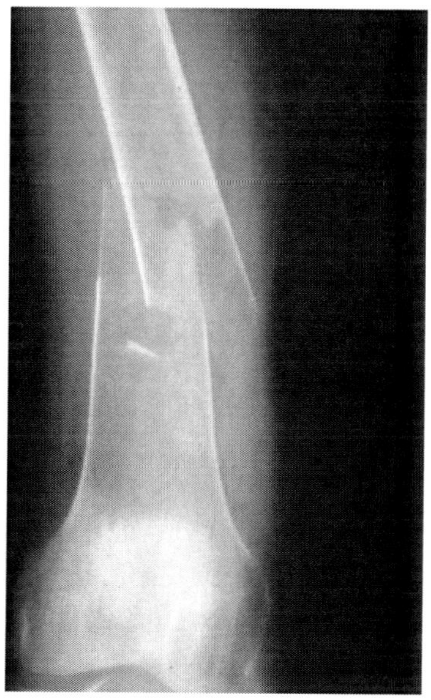

Figure 1. Spontaneous fracture of the distal right femur in a 74-year-old woman who was being lifted onto a operating table after a fracture of the proximal left femur. This was the first indication that she had severe osteomalacia; her serum 25OHD was 1.5 ng/mL.

**Table 1. Causes of fractures or of a significantly low bone density in patients referred for osteoporosis assessment to one clinic over four years [17]**

| | Number of patients | | |
|---|---|---|---|
| | **Men** | **Women** | **Total** |
| Osteoporosis (no cause found) | 13 | 128 | 141 |
| Osteomalacia* | 2 | 28 | 30 |
| Coeliac disease without osteomalacia | 0 | 3 | 3 |
| Hypogonadism | 16 | 3 | 19 |
| Osteogenesis imperfecta | 1 | 4 | 5 |
| Paraproteinaemia or lymphoma | 0 | 4 | 4 |

* Including two men and nine women found to have malabsorption.

In the clinical assessment of patients found to have osteomalacia history taking should include questions related to vitamin D intake, such as on diet and sunlight exposure, and questions related to possible underlying causes of deficiency, such as malabsorption or liver disease.

## Clinical Examination

Bone tenderness is a useful pointer to osteomalacia in some patients. It is elicited by gentle pressure on the rib cage or pelvis. Muscle weakness may be demonstrated by difficulty in getting out of a chair or getting up from a lying position.

## Clinical Biochemistry

About two thirds of patients with osteomalacia have hypocalcaemia and a similar proportion have a low serum inorganic phosphate. Most patients have a raised serum alkaline phosphatase but it is important to recognise that high values have a substantial differential diagnosis. This includes Paget's disease of bone, obstructive liver disease and pregnancy (placental alkaline phosphatase). When osteomalacia is treated with vitamin D the serum alkaline phosphatase often rises substantially before falling towards normal.

The most useful biochemical investigations for osteomalacia are serum 25-hydroxyvitamin D (25OHD) and serum parathyroid hormone (PTH). There are considerable difficulties in the interpretation of 25OHD values. The identification of a reference range in the conventional way (as 95% of a normal population) is not appropriate since in any country the values in the general population depend on the habitual lifestyle and diet. In addition, even in western countries, there are appreciable numbers of asymptomatic individuals who are, in fact, deficient.

One way round this problem is to regard as abnormal values below which the serum PTH is often raised. In one study [18] the value was 37 nmol/L (15 ng/mL). Another approach is to identify serum 25 OHD levels below which fracture risk is increased. In one study of older men [19] this was 40 nmol/L (16 ng/mL). Fuller accounts of the difficulties in defining reference ranges for serum 25OHD are provided elsewhere [20-22]. In addition the analytical results depend in part on the choice of assay [20, 23, 24].

In most patients with symptomatic osteomalacia 25OHD values are below 25 nmol/L (10 ng/mL). There is some indications that 25OHD values between 25 and 50 nmol/L (10 and 20 ng/mL) may be detrimental in other ways. Some of the evidence for this depends on associations between non-bone conditions and moderately low serum 25OHD levels and remains controversial [19, 21, 25]. A raised serum or plasma PTH is a sensitive pointer to secondary hyperparathyroidism and useful in supporting the diagnosis of vitamin D deficiency. A variety of different methods are available and the quoted reference ranges vary appreciably. The appropriateness of these reference values depends in part on the population used to define them [26].

In oncogenic osteomalacia and in most cases of heritable hypophosphataemia the blood FGF23 is greatly raised. It is important to be aware of the technical difficulties with this assay; serum is not satisfactory unless rapidly frozen and EDTA plasma is preferable [27].

# Radiology

Most patients with osteomalacia have no radiological abnormality. Overt osteopenia is uncommon. A few patients present with fractures and a few have pseudofractures (Looser zones, Milkman fractures). These can be distinguished from true fractures by the lack of local physical signs; there is no histological discontinuity. In addition, the radiological appearances of pseudofractures do not change until vitamin D replacement is started. Examples of pseudofractures are shown in figures 2, 3 and 4.

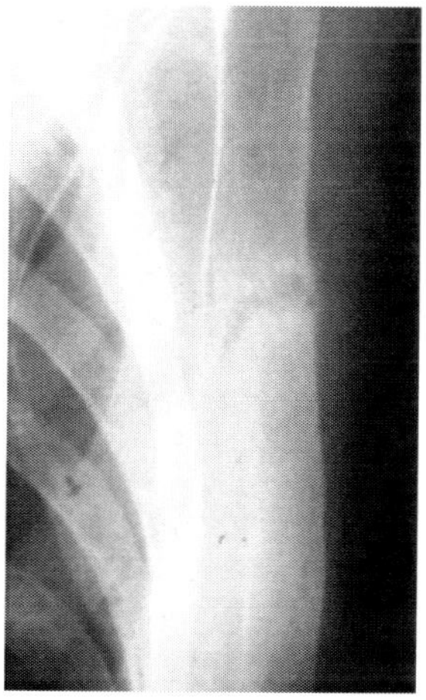

Figure 2. Pseudofracture of scapula in a woman with post-gastrectomy osteomalacia.

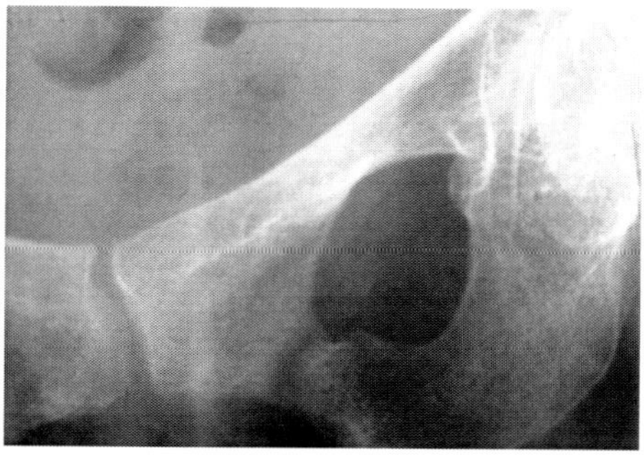

Figure 3. Pseudofracture of pelvis in a 65-year-old woman with post-gastrectomy osteomalacia. She had had symptoms of bone pain, fractures and muscle weakness for four years before the diagnosis was made.

While pseudofractures are interesting findings and helpful in supporting the diagnosis of osteomalacia the use of extensive radiology to search for pseudofractures cannot be justified at a time when biochemical investigation is much more relevant.

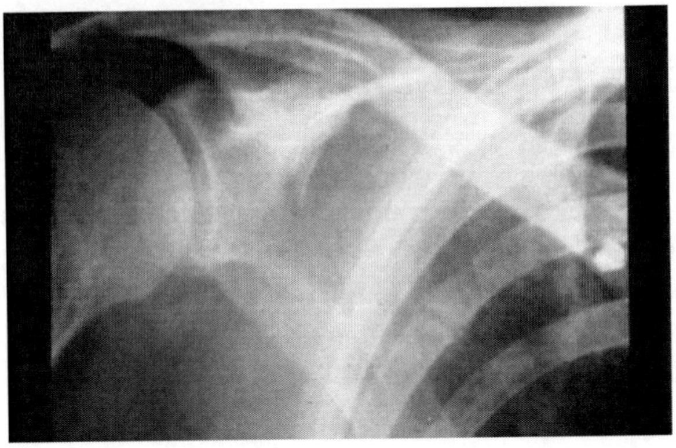

Figure 4. Pseudofracture of rib in a woman with nutritional osteomalacia.

## Densitometry

While low values after bone densitometry may be the first pointer to a diagnosis of osteomalacia it is important to recognise that not all patients have values outside the reference range. In one recent study [28] only 70% of the patients had T-scores lower than minus three. The lack of osteopenia does not exclude osteomalacia.

Densitometry may be helpful in demonstrating a response to treatment with vitamin D and very large improvements are seen particularly at sites assessing trabecular bone [29]. Similar striking increases have been seen after appropriate treatment in hypophosphataemic osteomalacia [30].

## Scintigraphy

Bone scanning with Tc99m to demonstrate areas of increased bone blood flow are valuable for example in a search for secondary neoplasm. Since the symptoms of osteomalacia and of skeletal secondaries may be similar, isotope bone scans may be undertaken. In a few patients with osteomalacia the fractures and pseudofractures may lead to appearances that mimic multiple deposits (figure 5). Similar cases of misdiagnosis have been reported by others [32].

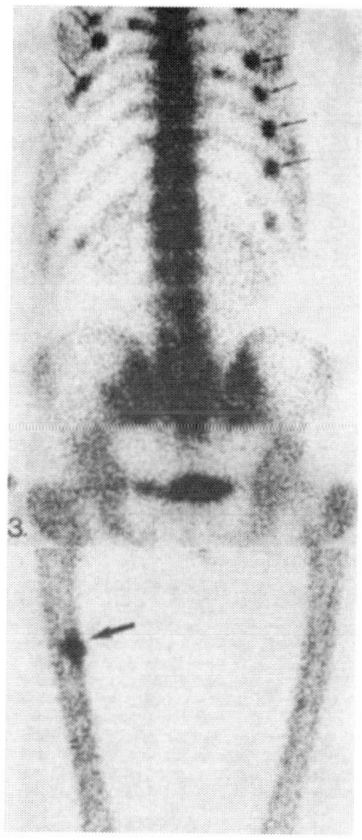

Figure 5. Multiple areas of increased uptake on Tc 99m bone scanning in a 73-year-old woman admitted for the investigation of bone pain and inability to walk. Secondary neoplasm was considered possible and a bone scan was requested. The appearances were thought more consistent with osteomalacia; she was treated with calciferol and within three weeks she was again able to walk.

Occasionally bone scintigraphy may demonstrate the site of the causative tumour in oncogenic osteomalacia [33].

# Bone Biopsy

At one time bone biopsy, generally of trabecular bone of the iliac crest, was regarded as essential for the objective diagnosis of osteomalacia. It was important to be able to prepare sections of undecalcified bone and so to assess the amount of uncalcified bone matrix or osteoid. The need for bone biopsy was questioned as early as 1993 [34]. With the availability of modern biochemical tests of serum 25OHD and parathyroid hormone, bone biopsy can nowadays seldom be justified.

# Response to Treatment

Osteomalacia is a most satisfactory disorder to treat. The administration of vitamin D in deficient cases leads to an improvement in the bone pain in about two weeks. The biochemical abnormalities improve more slowly and the bone density more gradually still. The symptoms of patients with hereditary hypophosphataemic osteomalacia and of oncogenic osteomalacia improve with calcitriol and phosphate supplements. Oncogenic osteomalacia is cured if the underlying tumour can be identified and removed.

## Acknowledgments

I thank Mrs. Sally Paterson for her help in all stages of the preparation of this review,

## References

[1] Maxwell, JP; Pi, HT; Lin, HAC; Kuo, CC. Further studies in adult rickets (osteomalacia) and foetal rickets. *Proc Roy Soc Med*, 1939, 32, 287-97.

[2] Holick, MF; Chen, TC. Vitamin D deficiency: a worldwide problem with health consequences. *Am J Clin Nutr*, 2008, 87 (suppl), 1080S–6S.

[3] Palacios, C; Gonzalez, L. Is vitamin D deficiency a major global public health problem? *J Steroid Biochem Mol Biol*, 2014, 144A, 138-45.

[4] Macdonald, HM; Mavroeidi, A; Fraser, WD; et al. Sunlight and dietary contributions to the seasonal vitamin D status of cohorts of healthy postmenopausal women living at northerly latitudes: a major cause for concern? *Osteoporos Int*, 2011, 22, 2461-72.

[5] Paterson, CR. Osteomalacia after partial gastrectomy: the time-scale of vitamin D depletion. In *Clinical Aspects of Metabolic Bone Disease* (1973) ed. Frame B, Parfitt AM and Duncan H, p380, Amsterdam: Excerpta Medica.

[6] Burns, J; Paterson, CR. Single dose vitamin D treatment for osteomalacia in the elderly. *Br Med J*, 1985, 290, 281-2.

[7] Bikle, DD. Vitamin D insufficiency/deficiency in gastrointestinal disorders. *J Bone Miner Res*, 2007, 22 (suppl 2), V50-4.

[8] Chong, WH; Molinolo, AA; Chen, CC; Collins, MT. Tumor-induced osteomalacia. *Endocr Relat Cancer*, 2011, 18, R53-77.

[9] Jiang, Y; Xia, WB; Xing, XP; et al. Tumor-induced osteomalacia: an important cause of adult-onset hypophosphatemic osteomalacia in China: report of 39 cases and review of the literature. *J Bone Miner Res*, 2012, 27, 1967-75.

[10] Jeong, HJ; Lee, JM; Lee, TH; et al. Two cases of hypophosphatemic osteomalacia after long-term low dose adefovir therapy in chronic hepatitis B and literature review. *J Bone Metab*, 2014, 21, 76-83.

[11] Nellen, JFJB; Smulders, YM; Jos, Frissen, PH; Slaats, EH; Silverbusch, J. Hypovitaminosis D in immigrant women: slow to be diagnosed. *BMJ*, 1996, 312, 570-2.

[12] Ralston, SH; Willocks, L; Pitkeathly, DA; Morton, R; Smith, GD. High prevalence of unrecognized osteomalacia in hospital patients with rheumatoid arthritis. *Br J Rheumatol*, 1988, 27, 202-5.

[13] Al Allaf, AW; Mole, PA; Paterson, CR; Pullar, T. Bone health in patients with fibromyalgia. *Rheumatology*, 2003, 42, 1202-6.

[14] Bours, SP; van Geel, TA; Geusens, PP; et al. Contributors to secondary osteoporosis and metabolic bone diseases in patients presenting with a clinical fracture. *J Clin Endocrinol Metab*, 2011, 96, 1360-7.

[15] Brinker, MR; O'Connor, DP; Monla, YT; Earthman, TP. Metabolic and endocrine abnormalities in patients with nonunions. *J Orthop Trauma*, 2007, 21, 557-70.

[16] Herm, FB; Killguss, H; Stewart, AG. Osteomalacia in Hazara District, Pakistan. *Trop Doct*, 2005, 35, 8-10.
[17] Paterson, CR; Mole, PA; Wilson, SJ. Osteopenia has a differential diagnosis. *Scott Med J*, 2001, 46, 163-4.
[18] Thomas, MK; Lloyd-Jones, DM; Thadhani, RI; et al. Hypovitaminosis D in medical inpatients. *N Engl J Med*, 1998, 338, 777-83.
[19] Rosen, CJ. Vitamin D insufficiency. *N Engl J M*ed, 2011, 364, 248-54.
[20] Krasowski, MD. Pathology consultation on vitamin D testing. *Am J Clin Pathol*, 2011, 136, 507-14.
[21] Harvey, NC; Cooper, C. Vitamin D: some perspective please. *BMJ*, 2012, 345, e4695.
[22] Shaw, NJ; Mughal, MZ. Vitamin D and child health: part 2 (extraskeletal and other aspects). *Arch Dis Child*, 2013, 98, 368-72.
[23] Snellman, G; Melhus, H; Gedeborg, R; et al. Determining vitamin status: a comparison between commercially available assays. *Plos One*, 2010, 5, e11555.
[24] Lai, JKC; Lucas, RM; Clements, MS; Harrison, SL; Banks, E. Assessing vitamin D status: pitfalls for the unwary. *Mol Nutr Food Res*, 2010, 54, 1062-71.
[25] Welsh, P; Peters, MJL; Sattar, N. Vitamin D insufficiency. *N Engl J Med*, 2011, 364, 1378-9.
[26] Deckers, MML; de Jongh, RT; Lips, PTAM; et al. Prevalence of vitamin D deficiency and consequences for PTH reference values. *Clin Chim Acta*, 2013, 426, 41-5.
[27] Mayo Medical Laboratories. Fibroblast growth factor 23 (FGF23), plasma. http://www.mayomedicallaboratories.com/ test-catalog/ Clinical + and + interpretative / 88662.
[28] Saghafi, M; Azarian, A; Hashemzadeh, K; Sahebari, M; Rezaieyazdi, Z. Bone densitometry in patients with osteomalacia, is it valuable? *Clin Cases Miner Bone Metab*, 2013, 10, 180-2.
[29] Bhambri, R; Naik, V; Malhotra, N; et al. Changes in bone mineral density following treatment of osteomalacia. *J Clin Densitom*, 2006, 9, 120-7.
[30] Negri, AL; Bogado, CE; Zanchetta, JR. Bone densitometry in a patient with hypophosphatemic osteomalacia. *J Bone Miner Metab*, 2004, 22, 514-7.
[31] Paterson, CR; Hadden, WA; Neill, GDS. Radionuclide bone scans in osteomalacia mimic those of malignant disease. *J Neurol Orthop Med Surg*, 1988, 9, 57-9.
[32] Sievenpiper, JL; McIntyre, EA; Verrill, M; Quinton, R; Pearce, SHS. Unrecognised severe vitamin D deficiency. *BMJ*, 2008, 336, 1371-4.
[33] Palaniswamy, SS; Subramanyam, P; Kumar, H. Oncogenic osteomalacia diagnosed by blood pool scintigraphy. *Indian J Nucl Med*, 2011, 26, 188-91.
[34] Bingham, CT; Fitzpatrick, LA. Noninvasive testing in the diagnosis of osteomalacia. *Am J Med*, 1993, 95, 519-23.

In: Bone Disorders, Screening and Treatment
Editor: Aubrey M. Stone
ISBN: 978-1-63482-155-1


*Chapter 9*

# Osteomalacic Myopathy

***Ripellino Paolo*[*], *Comi Cristoforo, Mazzini Letizia and Cantello Roberto***
Department of Neurology, University of Eastern Piedmont, Novara, Italy

## Abstract

Osteomalacia is the equivalent of rickets in the adult and is due to severe, prolonged vitamin D depletion. The diagnosis is challenging and underestimated, but should be considered in patients suffering from proximal muscle weakness, bone pain and a gait disorder that leads to repeated falls. In the following chapter we present the clinical features of osteomalacic myopathy, we discuss current hypothesis about pathogenesis and we show muscle biopsy pictures and EMG recordings of a case recently diagnosed in our Department.

Our goal is to make physicians aware of this treatable condition to avoid misdiagnosis.

## Background

Osteomalacia is the equivalent of rickets in the adult and is caused by severe and prolonged (usually for years) vitamin D depletion. In developed countries the main causes of osteomalacia are related to acquired malabsorption [1], previous gastrectomy [2-8] for tumor removal or for bariatric surgery, and kidney failure with secondary hyperparathyroidism.

Osteomalacia is most common in elderly people, but insufficient sun exposure related to religious habits of integral coverage of the body with black clothes account for many cases among young women in the Middle-East, whereas malnutrition remains the main risk factor in undeveloped countries [9].

[*] pao.ripe@hotmail.it

The clinical picture seems nowadays so unusual that general practitioners may underestimate the symptoms, diagnosing "fibromyalgia" or recurring to expensive exams to exclude bone metastases as the cause of bone pain. However, in the worst scenario an untreatable neuromuscular disorder is diagnosed [10], with important clinical consequences for the patient, because the symptoms of osteomalacia are indeed manageable with appropriate vitamin supplementation.

# Physiology of Vitamin D on Muscle

The main studies on osteomalacia were performed in the 1970s and were focused only on bone metabolism [11-14].

More than 40 years ago, scientists tried to define the role of vitamin D in muscle metabolism with animal models. The soleus muscle of a rat deprived of vitamin D showed a prolonged relaxation phase, suggesting a sequester of calcium in the sarcoplasmic reticulum [15].

Smith and Stern [11], based on clinical observations on 45 patients with osteomalacia, could not find any relation between serum calcium level and the development of myopathy and therefore suggested hypophosphatemia as the main cause of mitochondrial dysfunctions. Indeed, rachitic rats with vitamin D and phosphate deficiency had muscle weakness, but this was reversible when vitamin D treatment significantly raised serum phosphorus levels to normal range [16].

It later became clear that vitamin D plays a role in other physiological functions such as muscle strength, cognitive performances and immune system regulation. Today the effect of vitamin D on muscle seems to be not only calcium- and phosphate-mediated (indirect), but also direct through a vitamin D receptor (VDR) [17, 18] that might regulate calcium metabolism and muscle cells proliferation. Since vitamin D acts as a steroid hormone, it could induce transcription of proteins involved in calcium metabolism [19-23].

## Clinical Presentation

Osteomalacia is a rare endocrine myopathy [24] with a chronic, slowly progressive course. The main clinical features are diffuse bone pain [14, 25, 26] worsened by digital pressure and bone tenderness that accounts for skeletal deformities as kyphoscolyosis and pseudofractures. In the past, bone biopsy was required to confirm the diagnosis [27], but nowadays bone alterations are well documentable by X-rays (figure 1) and by bone densitometry scan.

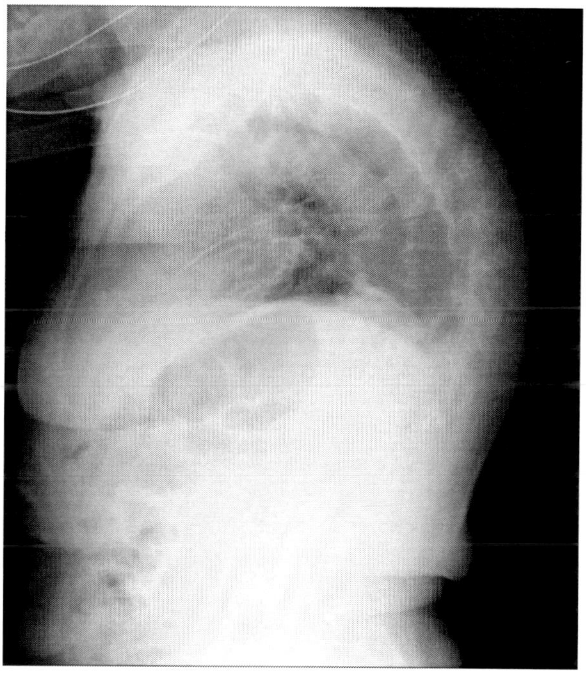

Figure 1. Chest x-ray of a patient with osteomalacic myopathy shows severe kyphoscoliosis.

Deep tendon reflexes are typically normal or brisk. Muscle atrophy and proximal limb muscle weakness [26, 28] cause difficulty in rising from a chair and walking up stairs. However, the degree of weakness might be difficult to assess because of coincidental bone pain. The altered balance [29] and the waddling gait (i.e., inability to lift the leg off the ground because of quadriceps weakness) may eventually contribute to the fear of falling [30] and to the real increased risk of fall of patients with severe vitamin D depletion [29].

In other words, among elderly patients the levels of vitamin D seem to be inversely associated with the risk of falling [31]. Several intervention trials in old patients with low vitamin D status have led to the conclusion that vitamin D supplementation improves muscle strength and balance [32-34].

A recent meta-nalysis [35] compared the results of daily vitamin D administration (800-1000 IU) among over 60 aged people, revealing that balance and muscle strength improved slightly, but the benefits on rate of falls seem to be greater in individuals who already have at baseline low serum levels of vitamin D.

## Laboratory Tests

The threshold for vitamin D deficiency is considered <30ng/ml, but in its classic presentation osteomalacia is associated with undetectable (<4 ng/ml) level of serum vitamin D, hypocalcemia, hypophosphatemia [36], and increased serum alkaline phosphatase. As a result of chronic hypocalcemia, serum parathormone (PTH) level increases, leading to bone reabsorption, reduced calcium and phosphate urinary levels [11, 27], increased phosphaturia **(table 1).** Creatinkinase (CK) level is usually normal, despite the majority of myopathies, and does not correlate with the degree of muscle weakness. Pancytopenia, probably related to PTH toxicity, may be observed in severe cases [37].

**Table 1.**

| | Laboratory test | Other suggested exams |
|---|---|---|
| FIRST LEVEL | B12, folic acid, vitamin D, parathormone (PTH), alkaline phosphatase (ALP), ionized calcium | X-rays |
| SECOND LEVEL | Phosphatemia, urinary calcium/24h, urinary phosphatum/24 h | EMG |
| THIRD LEVEL | | Muscle biopsy<br>Gastroscopy and investigation of malabsorption |

## Neurophysiology

Electrodiagnostic studies in osteomalacic myopathy [38, 39] usually show normal nerve conductions, but patients with concomitant malabsorption of other vitamins (mainly of the B complex and liposoluble) may suffer from associated polyneuropathy. Needle electromyography (EMG) examination must include proximal and distal muscles and may evidence normal findings or unspecific signs of chronic myopathy in more severely affected patients. Upper and lower limb-girdle muscles (e.g., deltoid and quadriceps femoris, respectively) examination at rest may show signs of chronic denervation as complex repetitive discharges (CRD). On voluntary contraction there is a combination of motor unit action potentials (MUAPs) typically myopathic, i.e. polyphasic with short duration and low amplitude, with MUAPs that are more commonly associated to neuropathic disorders, i.e. with long-duration, high-amplitude and polyphasic. The recruitment can be normal, early or slightly reduced.

## Histology

Muscle biopsy should be considered as a second level exam needed in case of uncertain diagnosis, for example if a paraneoplastic inflammatory myopathy has been suspected. Light microscopy shows unspecific findings such as fatty infiltration, interstitial fibrosis, sarcolemmal nuclear proliferation [40]. Some cases show selective type-II fiber atrophy [26, 29, 41] (figure 2a, 2b) that may be either explained by muscle disuse and/or by the selective expression of VDR on this type of fibers [18], rich in mitochondria and involved in fast twitching and in balance.

Indeed, mitochondria accumulate in the subsarcolemmal space (figure 2c) and areas devoid of nicotinamide adenine dinucleotide (NADH) [41] can be recognized within the muscle fibre. Type II fibres are efficient for short bursts of speed and power, but develop fatigue quicker. Their different metabolism can be visualized by dark brown staining in the ATPase staining at pH 9.4, whereas type I fibres appear lighter (figure 2b).

In a series of 10 patients, electronic microscopy detected loss of myofibrils, prominence of mitochondria and glycogen, loosening of the basement-membrane but preservation of myofibrils [42]. Similar findings in addition to adipose tissue deposition have been reported also by other authors [38, 43, 44].

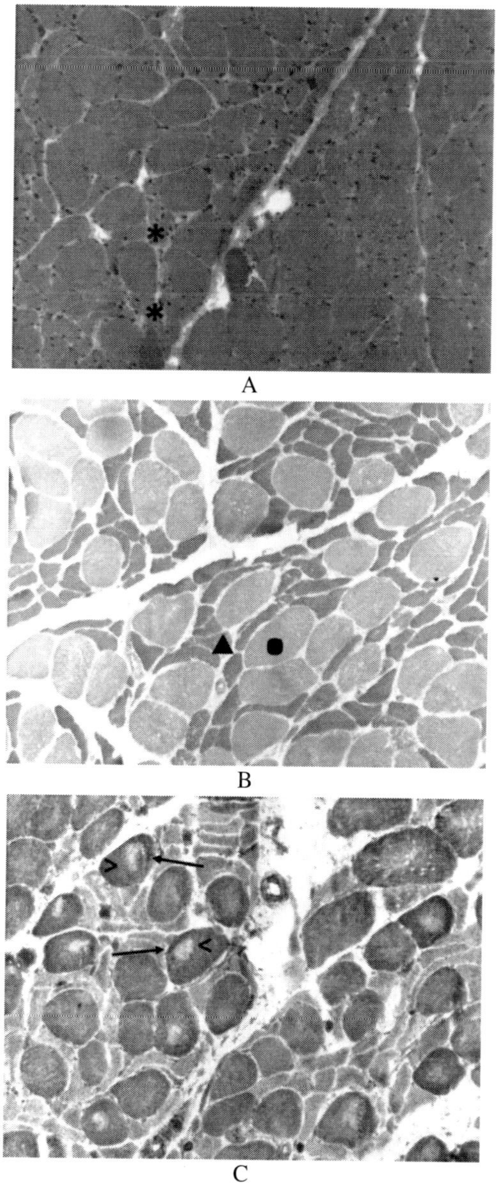


Figure 2. Biopsy of the right vastus lateralis muscle. A) Haematoxylin and eosin (H&E) staining at 100x shows type II fibre atrophy (asterisk), as confirmed in B) with the ATPase pH 9.4 staining at 100x. Type II fibres, rich of mitochondria, appear dark brown stained (triangle), whereas type I fibres are light brown (circle). C) NADH staining at 100x shows fibres devoid of oxidative activity (arrowheads) and subsarcolemmal accumulation of mitochondria (arrows).

Sato and colleagues studied in a randomized controlled trial [29] the effect of vitamin D supplementation in elderly stroke patients with hemiplegia. Patients were biopsied in the not paralyzed vastus lateralis muscle at baseline and after 2 years of supplementation vitamin D 1000 UI/daily). The initial type II fibre atrophy was reversible and the rate of falls in the treated group was 60% less.

### Treatment

All myopathic symptoms are fully reversible after vitamin D and calcium supplementation [30, 45]. Combined calcium and vitamin D oral treatment leads after few weeks to bone pain disappearance, muscle strength improvement [14, 30] , as well as changes in the EMG recordings (video).

## References

[1] Basha B, Rao DS, Han ZH, Parfitt AM. Osteomalacia due to vitamin D depletion: a neglected consequence of intestinal malabsorption. *Am. J Med.* Mar 2000;108(4):296-300.

[2] Kikuchi H, Ujiie S, Kanamaru R. Osteomalacia that became symptomatic 13 years after a total gastrectomy. *Intern. Med.* May 2000;39(5):394-396.

[3] Folli F, Sabowitz BN, Schwesinger W, Fanti P, Guardado-Mendoza R, Muscogiuri G. Bariatric surgery and bone disease: from clinical perspective to molecular insights. *International Journal of Obesity.* 2012;36(11):1373-1379.

[4] Bisballe S, Eriksen EF, Melsen F, Mosekilde L, Sorensen OH, Hessov I. Osteopenia and osteomalacia after gastrectomy: interrelations between biochemical markers of bone remodelling, vitamin D metabolites, and bone histomorphometry. *Gut.* Nov 1991;32(11):1303-1307.

[5] Morgan DB, Paterson CR, Woods CG, Pulvertaft CN, Fourman P. Search for osteomalacia in 1228 patients after gastrectomy and other operations on the stomach. *Lancet.* Nov 27 1965;2(7422):1085-1088.

[6] Morgan DB, Paterson CR, Woods CG, Pulvertaft CN, Fourman P. Osteomalacia after gastrectomy. A response to very small doses of vitamin D. *Lancet.* Nov 27 1965;2(7422):1089-1091.

[7] Morgan DB, Pulvertaft CN, Fourman P. Effects of age on the loss of bone after gastric surgery. *Lancet.* Oct 8 1966;2(7467):772-773.

[8] Bisballe S, Buus S, Lund B, Hessov I. Food intake and nutritional status after gastrectomy. *Hum. Nutr. Clin. Nutr.* Jul 1986;40(4):301-308.

[9] Haroon M, Regan MJ. Vitamin D deficiency: the time to ignore it has passed. *Int. J. Rheum. Dis.* Oct 2010;13(4):318-323.

[10] Muthukrishnan J, Harikumar KV, Sangeeta J, Singh MK, Modi K. Nerve, muscle or bone disease? Look before you leap. *Singapore Med. J.* Aug 2009;50(8):e293-294.

[11] Smith R, Stern G. Myopathy, osteomalacia and hyperparathyroidism. *Brain.* Sep 1967;90(3):593-602.

[12] Mankin HJ. Rickets, osteomalacia, and renal osteodystrophy. Part II. *J. Bone Joint Surg. Am.* Mar 1974;56(2):352-386.

[13] Mankin HJ. Rickets, osteomalacia, and renal osteodystrophy. An update. *Orthop Clin North Am.* Jan 1990;21(1):81-96.

[14] Schott GD, Wills MR. Myopathy in hypophosphataemic osteomalacia presenting in adult life. *J. Neurol. Neurosurg. Psychiatry.* Mar 1975;38(3):297-304.

[15] Rodman JS, Baker T. Changes in the kinetics of muscle contraction in vitamin D-depleted rats. *Kidney Int.* Mar 1978;13(3):189-193.

[16] Schubert L, DeLuca HF. Hypophosphatemia is responsible for skeletal muscle weakness of vitamin D deficiency. *Arch. Biochem. Biophys.* Aug 15 2010;500(2):157-161.

[17] Simpson RU, Thomas GA, Arnold AJ. Identification of 1,25-dihydroxyvitamin D3 receptors and activities in muscle. *J. Biol. Chem.* Jul 25 1985;260(15):8882-8891.

[18] Bischoff HA, Borchers M, Gudat F, et al. In situ detection of 1,25-dihydroxyvitamin D3 receptor in human skeletal muscle tissue. *Histochem J.* Jan 2001;33(1):19-24.

[19] Ceglia L. Vitamin D and skeletal muscle tissue and function. *Molecular Aspects of Medicine.* 2008;29(6):407-414.

[20] Ceglia L, Harris SS. Vitamin D and Its Role in Skeletal Muscle. *Calcified Tissue International.* 2012;92(2):151-162.

[21] Jones AN, Hansen KE. Recognizing the musculoskeletal manifestations of vitamin D deficiency. *J. Musculoskelet Med.* Oct 2009;26(10):389-396.

[22] Hamilton B. Vitamin D and human skeletal muscle. *Scand. J. Med. Sci. Sports.* Apr 2010;20(2):182-190.

[23] Birge SJ, Haddad JG. 25-hydroxycholecalciferol stimulation of muscle metabolism. *J. Clin. Invest.* Nov 1975;56(5):1100-1107.

[24] Kendall-Taylor P, Turnbull DM. Endocrine myopathies. *Br. Med. J. (Clin Res Ed).* Sep 10 1983;287(6394):705-708.

[25] Fabbriciani G, Pirro M, Leli C, et al. Diffuse Muscoskeletal Pain and Proximal Myopathy. *JCR: Journal of Clinical Rheumatology.* 2010;16(1):34-37.

[26] Russell JA. Osteomalacic myopathy. *Muscle Nerve.* Jun 1994;17(6):578-580.

[27] Reginato AJ, Falasca GF, Pappu R, McKnight B, Agha A. Musculoskeletal manifestations of osteomalacia: report of 26 cases and literature review. *Semin Arthritis Rheum.* Apr 1999;28(5):287-304.

[28] Schott GD, Wills MR. Muscle weakness in osteomalacia. *Lancet.* Mar 20 1976;1(7960):626-629.

[29] Sato Y, Iwamoto J, Kanoko T, Satoh K. Low-dose vitamin D prevents muscular atrophy and reduces falls and hip fractures in women after stroke: a randomized controlled trial. *Cerebrovasc Dis.* 2005;20(3):187-192.

[30] Ripellino P, Terazzi E, Bersano E, Cantello R. Adult osteomalacia: a treatable cause of "fear of falling" gait. *Neurology.* May 28 2013;80(22):2079.

[31] Snijder MB, van Schoor NM, Pluijm SM, van Dam RM, Visser M, Lips P. Vitamin D status in relation to one-year risk of recurrent falling in older men and women. *J. Clin. Endocrinol. Metab.* Aug 2006;91(8):2980-2985.

[32] Pfeifer M, Begerow B, Minne HW, Suppan K, Fahrleitner-Pammer A, Dobnig H. Effects of a long-term vitamin D and calcium supplementation on falls and parameters

of muscle function in community-dwelling older individuals. *Osteoporos. Int.* Feb 2009;20(2):315-322.

[33] Bischoff HA, Stahelin HB, Dick W, et al. Effects of vitamin D and calcium supplementation on falls: a randomized controlled trial. *J. Bone Miner Res.* Feb 2003;18(2):343-351.

[34] Dhesi JK, Jackson SH, Bearne LM, et al. Vitamin D supplementation improves neuromuscular function in older people who fall. *Age Ageing.* Nov 2004;33(6):589-595.

[35] Muir SW, Montero-Odasso M. Effect of vitamin D supplementation on muscle strength, gait and balance in older adults: a systematic review and meta-analysis. *J. Am. Geriatr. Soc.* Dec 2011;59(12):2291-2300.

[36] Mallette LE, Patten BM, Engel WK. Neuromuscular disease in secondary hyperparathyroidism. *Ann. Intern. Med.* Apr 1975;82(4):474-483.

[37] Lim DJ, Oh EJ, Park CW, et al. Pancytopenia and secondary myelofibrosis could be induced by primary hyperparathyroidism. *International Journal of Laboratory Hematology.* 2007;29(6):464-468.

[38] Floyd M, Ayyar DR, Barwick DD, Hudgson P, Weightman D. Myopathy in chronic renal failure. *Q. J. Med.* Oct 1974;43(172):509-524.

[39] Irani PF. Electromyography in nutritional osteomalacic myopathy. *J. Neurol Neurosurg Psychiatry.* Jul 1976;39(7):686-693.

[40] Skaria J, Katiyar BC, Srivastava TP, Dube B. Myopathy and neuropathy associated with osteomalacia. *Acta. Neurol. Scand.* Jan 1975;51(1):37-58.

[41] Palmucci L, Bertolotto A, Doriguzzi C, Mongini T, Coda R. Osteomalacic myopathy in a case of diffuse nodular lipomatosis of the small bowel. *Acta. Neurol. Belg.* Mar-Apr 1982;82(2):65-71.

[42] Dastur DK, Gagrat BM, Wadia NH, Desai M, Bharucha EP. Nature of muscular change in osteomalacia: light- and electron-microscope observations. *J. Pathol.* Dec 1975;117(4):211-228.

[43] Yoshikawa S, Nakamura T, Tanabe H, Imamura T. Osteomalacic myopathy. *Endocrinol. Jpn.* Jun 1979;26(Suppl):65-72.

[44] Lazaro RP, Kirshner HS. Proximal muscle weakness in uremia. Case reports and review of the literature. *Arch. Neurol.* Sep 1980;37(9):555-558.

[45] Al-Said YA, Al-Rached HS, Al-Qahtani HA, Jan MM. Severe proximal myopathy with remarkable recovery after vitamin D treatment. *Can. J. Neurol. Sci.* May 2009;36(3):336-339.

# Index

## A



## B

## C

## D



## E

## F



## G



## H

## I



## J



## K

## N



## O



## P

## Q



## R

## S



## T

## U



## V



## W

## X



## Y